Disorders of Steroidogenesis

Gill Rumsby • Gary M. Woodward
Editors

Disorders of Steroidogenesis

Guide to Steroid Profiling and Biochemical Diagnosis

Springer

Editors
Gill Rumsby
Department of Clinical Biochemistry
University College London Hospitals
London
UK

Gary M. Woodward
Department of Clinical Biochemistry
University College London Hospitals NHS
London
UK

ISBN 978-3-319-96363-1 ISBN 978-3-319-96364-8 (eBook)
https://doi.org/10.1007/978-3-319-96364-8

Library of Congress Control Number: 2018956736

This Springer imprint is published by the registered company Springer Nature Switzerland AG
The registered company address is: Gewerbestrasse 11, 6330 Cham, Switzerland

Preface

The diagnosis of disorders of steroidogenesis relies heavily on their biochemical investigations, with the most informative of these being the urine steroid profile. Urine steroid profiling by gas chromatography-mass spectrometry was first used in the 1970s and, even in these times of extensive use of liquid chromatography mass spectrometry (LCMS), the technique maintains its superiority as a means of comprehensively screening for a number of steroid disorders in a single test.

It was recognised that a loss of knowledge and expertise in the field of steroid disorders and urine steroid profiling was occurring through the retirement of key field leaders such as Gill Rumsby, John Honour, Norman Taylor and Cedric Shackleton. This motivated the initiation of this project, with the key aim of capturing knowledge and expertise that, up until now, has only been available in primary literature or anecdotally. What we have tried to achieve in this book is a compendium of the steroid disorders that are amenable to analysis by urine steroid profiling. This has built on the work of the only previously published reference text in this vein, written in 1981 (C.H.L. Shackleton, N.F. Taylor, J.W. Honour—*An Atlas of Gas Chromatographic Profiles of Neutral Urinary Steroids in Health and Disease*). In contrast to its predecessor and other titles on the topic of steroidogenic disorders, we offer a detailed review of each disorder, its biochemical and genetic features along with the characteristic metabolite findings, mass spectra and analytical pitfalls. It can therefore provide a revision primer for these disorders as well as a manual for urine steroid profiling.

We hope we have achieved this aim.

London, UK — Gill Rumsby
London, UK — Gary M. Woodward

Contents

Overview of Adrenal Physiology and Steroid Biochemistry

1

Gary M. Woodward and Gill Rumsby

1.1 Introduction

The investigation and diagnosis of adrenal steroidogenic conditions require knowledge of the chemistry and biochemistry of steroids along with an understanding of their physiological and clinical contexts. In the following chapters, a description of the relevant aspects of steroidogenesis and steroid metabolism will be reviewed in the context of normal physiology and pathology. As an introduction to this work, this chapter provides a simple account of steroid structure, chemistry and nomenclature, followed by a brief overview of the important aspects of steroid biosynthesis and metabolism. Throughout this chapter, reference will be made to an overriding concept that should be borne in mind throughout this text, namely, that steroidogenesis and metabolism are fundamentally different throughout the stages of human development.

1.1.1 Steroid Structures and Nomenclature

Steroids in their simplest form are organic compounds made up of a four-ring structure, A, B and C are cyclohexane rings, and D is a cyclopentane. These rings are arranged in a specific order to form the core steroid structure, known as a gonane or sterane. A hydroxyl on the A ring produces the basic sterol structure (Fig. 1.1).

The many different steroid species are defined and differentiated by functional groups, hydroxyl or carbon side chains, attached to the core sterol structure. Each carbon on the steroid structure is numbered according to the IUPAC atom numbering system as shown in Fig. 1.2.

G. M. Woodward (✉) · G. Rumsby
Department of Clinical Biochemistry, University College London Hospitals, London, UK
e-mail: Gary.Woodward1@nhs.net

G. Rumsby, G. M. Woodward (eds.), *Disorders of Steroidogenesis*,
https://doi.org/10.1007/978-3-319-96364-8_1

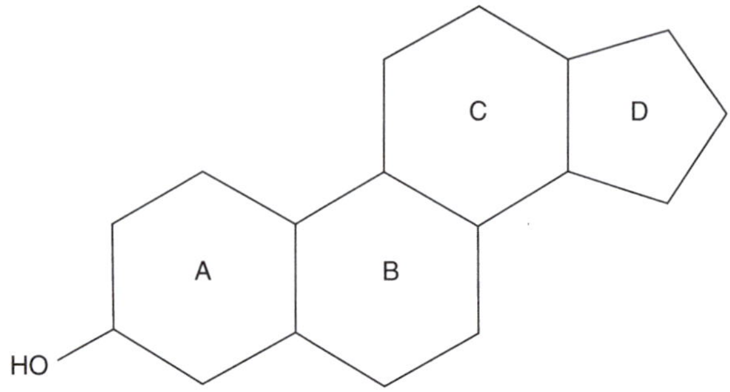

Fig. 1.1 Sterol structure

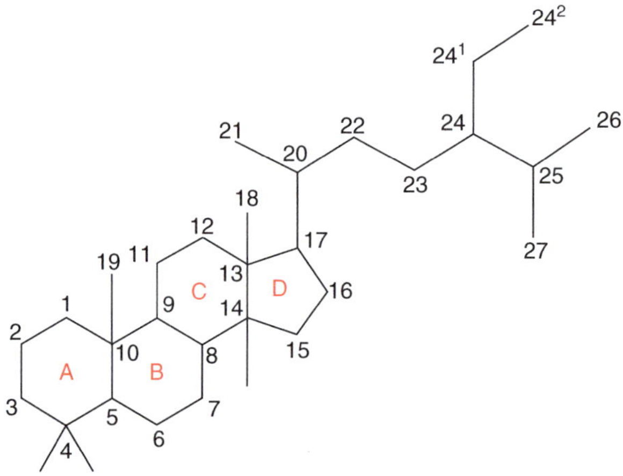

Fig. 1.2 Numbering of the steroid molecule based on IUPAC nomenclature

All steroids contain the first 17 carbons arranged to form continuous C–C bonds. The additional carbons 18–27 are steroid side chains. It is also important to bear in mind that the steroid structure may exist as one of two stereoisomeric forms, namely, α and β, that arise largely from the planar alignment of the hydrogen on carbon 5 of the A ring.

In addition to hydroxylation position and number, steroids may also vary in the bond orders within the rings, the number and position of methyl groups attached to the ring, the functional groups attached to the rings and in the configuration of groups attached to the rings. It should also be noted that steroid species may arise from cleavage (expansions and contractions) of the ring structure, such as that seen in vitamin D. However, in the context of adrenal steroidogenesis and metabolism, ring cleavage structures are not observed.

Adrenal or gonadal steroid species may be defined functionally into either corticosteroids or sex steroids. The corticosteroids (21 carbon steroids with a hydroxyl on the 21st carbon) consist of either glucocorticoids or mineralocorticoids. The sex steroids may be divided into progestogens (21 carbon structures, with no hydroxyl on the 21st carbon), oestrogens (18 carbon structures) or androgens (19 carbon structures).

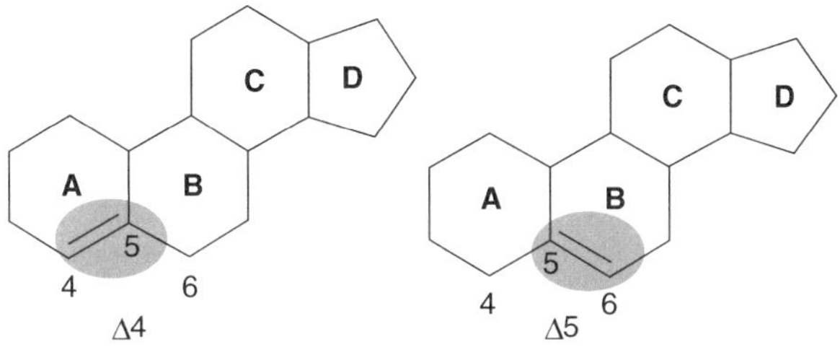

Fig. 1.3 Structural difference between delta 4 and 5 steroids

Throughout the literature and in clinical practice, specific steroid species may be referred to in many different ways. The International Union of Pure and Applied Chemistry (IUPAC) has commissioned a systematic nomenclature for naming and referring to steroids (*Pure & Appl. Chem. Vol 61 No 10 pp 1783–1822, 1989*). However, for ease and understanding, most refer to steroids by their common or trivial names or their abbreviations. For example, *11β,17,21-trihydroxypregn-4-ene3,20-dione* is the IUPAC name for cortisol that is also commonly abbreviated to compound F. Details of the common, abbreviated and IUPAC names for relevant steroids are shown in each chapter.

Steroids may also be referred to as either delta (Δ) 4 or Δ5 steroids. This refers to the possession and location of a double bond at carbons 4 or 5 of the steroid structure as shown in Fig. 1.3.

1.1.2 Structure and Function of the Adult Adrenal

The adult adrenal gland is made of two distinct parts, namely, the cortex and medulla. The main function of the adrenal cortex is to produce a variety of steroid hormones responsible for blood pressure regulation and electrolyte balance (mineralocorticoids), regulation of metabolism and immune system suppression (glucocorticoids) and extra-gonadal androgen production (particularly important in females). The cortex is comprised of three distinct zones, namely, the zona glomerulosa (ZG), zona reticularis (ZR) and zona fasciculata (ZF). The upper most layer (ZG) is made up of ovoid cells responsible for aldosterone production. The majority of the adrenal cortex is composed of the ZF, sitting just below the ZG, and is responsible for glucocorticoid production. The inner most layer of the adrenal cortex comprising the ZR is the site of adrenal androgen production.

While all the steroids produced in the adrenal are ultimately derived from cholesterol, distinct steroid structures result from each adrenal cortical zone as a function of their differential enzyme expressions. Aldosterone is the primary mineralocorticoid and is under the control of angiotensin II, forming part of the renin-angiotensin system. Ultimately aldosterone interacts with the nuclear mineralocorticoid receptor present in tissues including the colon, salivary gland and, most importantly, the renal distal convoluted tubule and collecting ducts. The main function of aldosterone is the reabsorption of sodium and increased excretion of both potassium and hydrogen ions. The ZF is the primary site for glucocorticoid production and is under the regulation of corticotrophic-releasing hormone (CRH) and adrenocorticotropic hormone (ACTH). Cortisol is the main glucocorticoid produced by the adrenal under normal conditions and serves to mobilise fats, proteins and carbohydrates, particularly during episodes of stress. The primary adrenal androgens produced by the ZR include dehydroepiandrosterone (DHEA) and androstenedione. These steroid species are converted in peripheral tissues to more potent androgens such as testosterone and play a role in androgen-sensitive hair growth. While the mechanism for adrenal androgen stimulation is still not completely described, ACTH stimulation plays a key role.

1.1.3 Steroid Synthesis

Steroid hormones are synthesised along a multi-enzymic pathway, sharing common precursors as illustrated in Fig. 1.4. The purpose of this complex pathway is the conversion of cholesterol to the major adrenal steroid hormones, cortisol, aldosterone and DHEA. The gonads are the major source of circulating androgens, progesterone, oestradiol and testosterone. The enzymes involved in steroid synthesis may be broadly grouped into two major classes: the cytochrome P450 haem-containing proteins (P450s) and the hydroxysteroid dehydrogenases (HSDs).

The P450s are membrane-bound proteins located either in the mitochondrion (CYP11A, CYP11B1, CYP11B2) or endoplasmic reticulum (CYP17, CYP19, CYP21), and all belong to a large family of haem-containing proteins that catalyse monooxygenase reactions (one atom of oxygen is inserted into the aliphatic position of an organic substrate, while the other oxygen atom is reduced to water). In relation

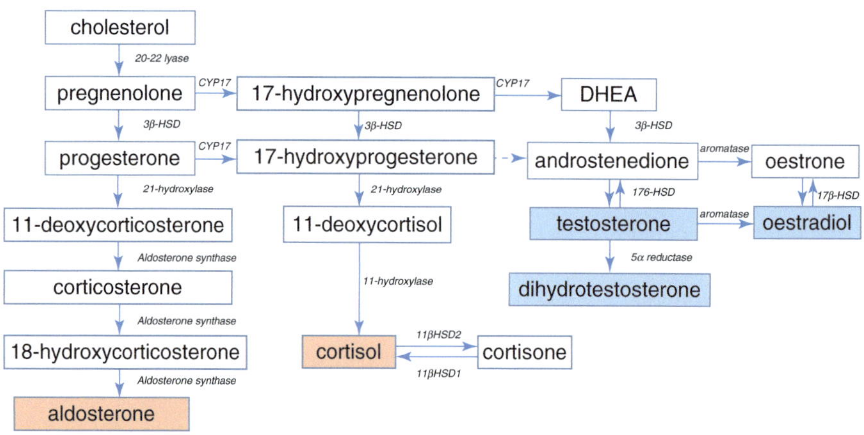

Fig. 1.4 Biosynthetic pathway for steroid hormones. The major adrenal steroids are highlighted in pink, gonadal steroids in blue. *DHEA* dehydroepiandrosterone, *3βHSD* 3β-hydroxysteroid dehydrogenase, *11βHSD* 11β-hydroxysteroid dehydrogenase, *17βHSD* 17β-hydroxysteroid dehydrogenase, *CYP17* 17α-hydroxylase

to steroid hormone synthesis, the P450 enzymes catalyse hydroxylation or cleavage reactions.

The first and rate limiting step in the conversion of cholesterol to steroid hormones is the hydroxylation of cholesterol on the C22 and C20 carbons. This reaction is catalysed by cholesterol side chain cleavage enzyme CYP11A1 (Fig. 1.5). The subsequent cleavage of the C22 and C20 hydroxyls results in the formation of the C21 steroid, pregnenolone. CYP11A1 is expressed in all three zones of the adrenal cortex as well as in gonadal and placental tissue and is expressed in the fetal adrenal from 14 to 23 weeks of gestation.

Pregnenolone (a Δ5 steroid) and progesterone (a Δ4 steroid) are hydroxylated on carbon C17 by the action of CYP17 to form 17α-hydroxypregnenolone (a Δ5 steroid) and 17α-hydroxyprogesterone (17OHP, a Δ4 steroid), respectively. These two 17-hydroxylated steroids may be thought of as intermediate steroid species as CYP17 subsequently catalyses the cleavage of the C17–20 bond, resulting in the formation of C19 steroids DHEA (a Δ5 steroid) and androstenedione (a Δ4 steroid), respectively, although the Δ5 steroid pathway is favoured in humans (Fig. 1.6).

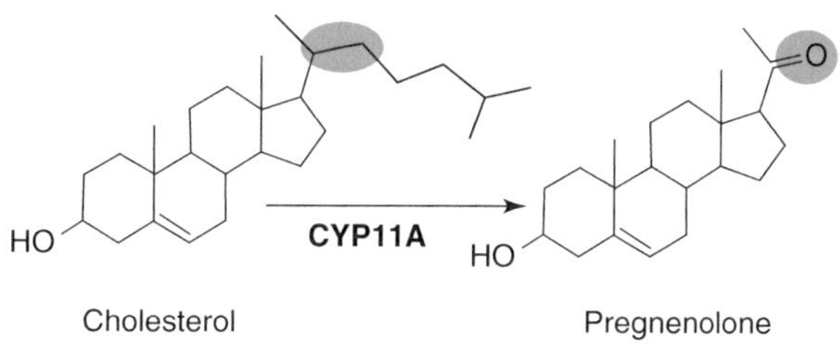

Fig. 1.5 Enzymatic reaction catalysed by cholesterol side-chain cleavage enzyme (CYP11A1)

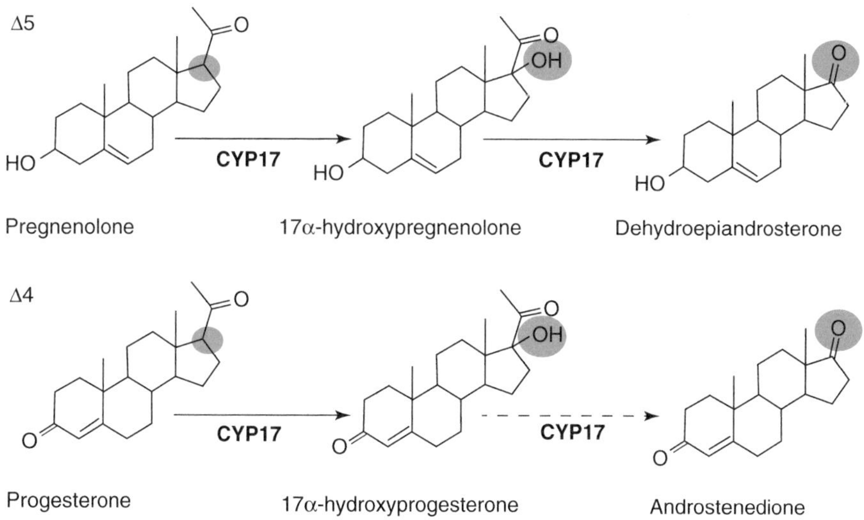

Fig. 1.6 Enzymatic reaction catalysed by 17α-hydroxylase (CYP17). 17OHP is a poor substrate for the enzyme in the human (see Chap. 7)

CYP17 is expressed in all steroidogenic tissues but not in all cell types, for example, within the adrenal, it is expressed within the ZR and ZF, but not in the ZG.

Hydroxylation of the Δ4 steroids progesterone and 17OHP is catalysed by CYP21 to form 11-deoxycorticosterone (DOC) and 11-deoxycortisol (also known as compound S), respectively (Fig. 1.7). Of note, hydroxylation of the progesterone by CYP21 occurs in the ZG that does not express CYP17. As such, 11-deoxycorticosterone cannot be converted to 11-deoxycortisol to produce cortisol. CYP21 is present in all zones of the adrenal cortex, although the ZG and ZF exhibit the highest expression with very little expressed in the ZR. CYP21 expression first occurs in the fetal zone (FZ) of the fetal adrenal at about 14 weeks of gestation.

The final steps in cortisol and aldosterone synthesis are achieved by CYP11B1 and CYP11B2, respectively. In the first instance, 11-deoxycorticosterone and 11-deoxycortisol are hydroxylated on C11 to form corticosterone (also known as compound B) and cortisol, respectively (Fig. 1.8). This reaction is catalysed by CYP11B1 in the ZR and CYP11B2 in the ZG, the latter enzyme also catalysing the 18-hydroxylation and oxidation steps to synthesise aldosterone. CYP11B1 and CYP11B2 are expressed only in the adrenal cortex, with CYP11B2 found exclusively in the ZG. It should be noted that the expression of CYP11B1 is severalfold higher than CYP11B2.

The conversion of the C19 steroids androstenedione and testosterone into the C18 oestrogens, oestrone and oestradiol, respectively, is catalysed by aromatase

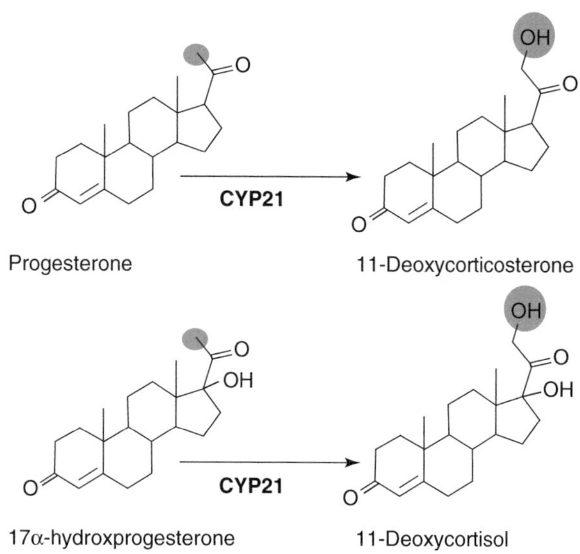

Fig. 1.7 Enzymatic reaction catalysed by 21-hydroxylase (CYP21)

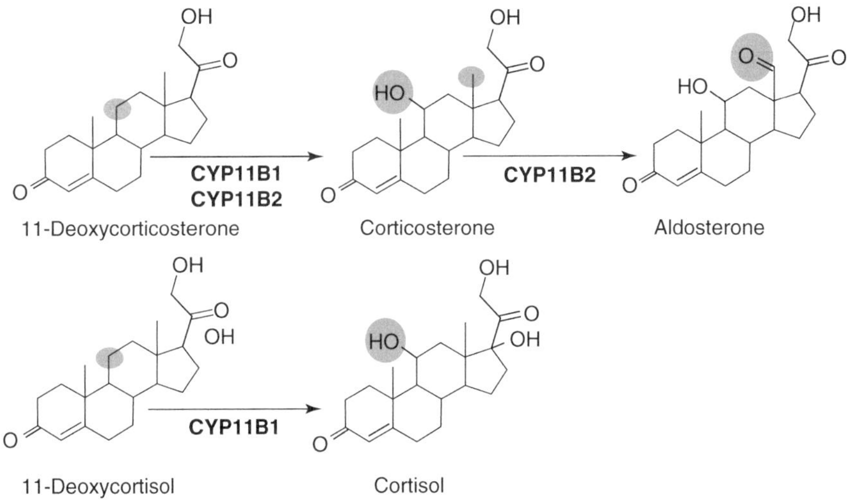

Fig. 1.8 Enzymatic reaction catalysed by 11β-hydroxylase (CYP11B1) and aldosterone synthase (CYP11B2)

(CYP19). This enzyme is not found in the adrenal but is found in the preovulatory follicle, corpus luteum, placenta and testicular tissue, particularly the interstitial tissue of the testes.

1.1.4 Hydroxysteroid Dehydrogenases

The hydroxysteroid dehydrogenases (HSDs) catalyse the reduction and oxidation of steroid hormones and belong to a family of short-chain alcohol dehydrogenase reductases. The biosynthesis of steroid hormones from Δ5-3-keto steroids to Δ4-3β-hydroxysteroids relies on the activity of 3βHSD, occurring as two isoforms, 3βHSD1 and 3βHSD2. The enzymes catalyse the conversion of pregnenolone, 17a-hydroxypregnenolone and DHEA to progesterone, 17OHP and androstenedione, respectively (Fig. 1.9). The 3βHSD2 is responsible for the majority of adrenal and gonadal steroid metabolism, while the 3βHSD1 isoform is expressed mainly in the placenta and peripheral tissues. Human 3βHSD expression occurs after week 23 of gestation in the fetal adrenal, but the fetus is unable to synthesise cortisol or aldosterone until late in gestation.

The final steps in gonadal steroidogenesis from androstenedione to testosterone and oestrone to oestradiol (Fig. 1.10) are catalysed by different isoenzymes of 17β-hydroxysteroid dehydrogenase (17βHSD).

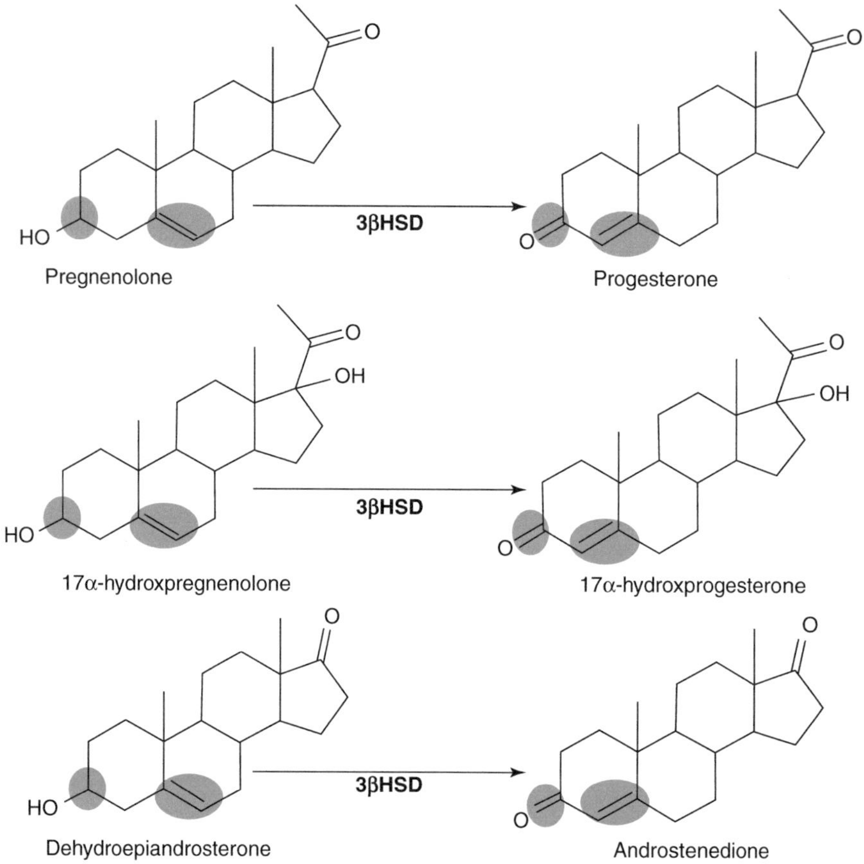

Fig. 1.9 Enzymatic reaction catalysed by 3β-hydroxysteroid dehydrogenase (3βHSD2)

1.2 The Fetal, Neonatal and Adolescent Adrenal

Many of the inborn errors of steroidogenesis present very early in life, usually the neonatal period. As such, it is important to bear in mind that the adrenal gland and its biochemistry are very different in the fetus, in the neonatal period and in adulthood. An understanding the steroid production in these periods is vital of the understanding and diagnosis of these early presenting diseases.

1.2.1 The Fetal Adrenal

The adrenal gland develops from two distinct embryological tissues, the adrenal medulla from neural crest cells and the cortex from the intermediate mesoderm. At about 30 days after conception, the adrenal gland begins to form as the

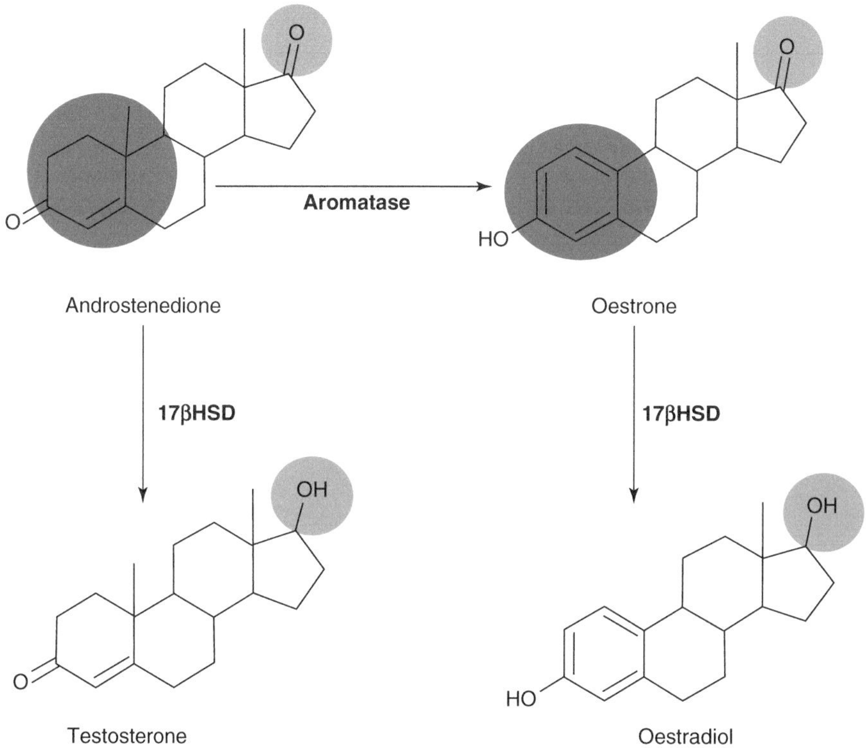

Fig. 1.10 Enzymatic reaction catalysed by different isoenzymes of 17β-hydroxysteroid dehydrogenase (17βHSD) and aromatase

adrenogonadal primordium (AGP). The AGP initially consists of a heterogeneous population of cells. Following a delamination event, most of the AGP cells migrate to form the gonadal primordial (GP), while a subset of AGP cells migrate to form the adrenal primordial (AP). The AP forms the early part of what later becomes the fetal adrenal. At about 48 days postconception, the neural crest cells (making up what becomes the adrenal medulla) migrate towards the AP. These cells remain scattered within the embryonic adrenal until differentiation into chromaffin cells to form the adrenal medulla after birth. These cells are responsible for catecholamine production.

The adrenal gland itself separates from its surrounding tissue (the mesenchyme) to become encapsulated by a layer of fibrous tissue. Cortical cells develop within the fibrous capsules until about day 52 postconception. After encapsulation, rapid expansion of the adrenal cortex occurs, where the enlarged fetal cortex makes up most of the prenatal adrenal growth, particularly in the last 6 weeks of gestation. The fetal zone (FZ) plays a major role in steroidogenesis at this time. It is relatively deficient in 3βHSD activity but expresses CYP17 with both 17 hydroxylase and 17,20 lyase activities, converting pregnenolone to DHEA and its sulphated metabolite, DHEAS, in large quantities. This steroid is then converted to oestrogens by the placenta to help maintain a normal pregnancy. In addition, large amounts of other Δ5 steroids are produced by the FZ, including pregnenolone and 17α-hydroxypregnenolone. These steroids occur mostly as sulphate conjugates.

Adrenocortical cells emerge between the capsule and FZ at about 8 weeks of gestation, forming a definitive zone that later develops into the adult cortex. As gestation progresses, the adrenocortical cells within the neocortex or definitive zone begin to expand, and by the third trimester, they produce cortisol under the regulation of ACTH. A concomitant ACTH-dependent increase in androstenedione and testosterone also takes place at this time. Cortisol production over this period then declines, while the production of DHEA predominates as described above. This early surge in cortisol production appears to be important in fetal adrenal regulation, and failure of this process, such as in CAH, results in overproduction of adrenal androgens and fetal virilisation.

The DAX1 gene (dosage-sensitive sex reversal, adrenal hypoplasia critical region, on chromosome X, gene 1, *NR0B1*) is of importance to the development of the adrenal cortex and primarily serves as a corepressor for steroidogenic factor 1 (SF1)-mediated transcription of steroidogenic genes. Regulation of DAX1 expression is dynamic and plays a key role in both the renewal of progenitor cells, adrenocortical differentiation and steroidogenesis in response to ACTH. In this regard, the growth and differentiation of the adrenal cortex are independent of ACTH stimulation during the first trimester, but it begins to play an important role after the 15th week of gestation. In late pregnancy, there is a steep increase in fetal cortisol production. While pituitary CRH is expressed throughout fetal and adult life, another important source of CRH is the placenta, and levels increase several 100-fold throughout gestation without causing excessive ACTH or cortisol synthesis in the mother or fetus—a mechanism that is not entirely understood. Placental CRH is thought to contribute to the induction of labour as well as glucose transport to the placenta and fetus. Placental CRH production may also stimulate cortisol production of fetal adrenocortical cells by upregulating the expression of steroidogenic acute regulatory protein and steroidogenic enzymes, including 3β-HSD2, CYP21 and CYP11B1. Another contributor to this process is likely to be placental and fetal 11β-HSD2 that rapidly metabolises cortisol to cortisone leading to enhanced clearance of cortisol that in turn promotes fetal ACTH stimulation of steroidogenesis.

1.2.2 The Neonatal Period

The neonatal period may be thought of as a dynamic transition between fetal and extrauterine life. It is also important to think of the neonate as not simply a miniature version of adult physiology but as discrete with its own characteristic physiology. This situation is particularly true for the adrenal, where steroid synthesis during the neonatal period is very different from that of the adult or, indeed, the fetus.

After birth, the fetal adrenal continues to undergo significant remodelling, first during the neonatal period to form a mature adrenal and during the early pubertal periods (adrenarche) to produce a competent adult adrenal. Fetal adrenal cells undergo apoptosis with concurrent maturation of the ZG and ZF under the drive of angiotensin II (AngII) and ACTH, respectively.

After birth, there is a decrease in cortisol production to a minimum at about 2 weeks of age, where it should remain stable. The cortisol response to stress is preserved in the neonate, and a diurnal rhythm has been seen as early as 3 days of age. The neonate exhibits high 11βHSD2 activity, and thus cortisol is rapidly metabolised to cortisone, but, with the loss of placental 11βHSD2, this situation is fairly rapidly replaced by the adult pattern where similar amounts of cortisol and cortisone metabolites are produced. The fetal zone steroids, predominantly Δ5 steroids, can persist for up to 6 months after birth particularly in premature infants. There is also significant activity of the 6α-hydroxylase enzyme leading to characteristic 6α-hydroxylated metabolites.

The fetal and neonatal adrenal are capable of converting corticosterone to aldosterone. Aldosterone production in late gestation and in the neonatal period is high due to a lack of mineralocorticoid receptor (MR) sensitivity in the neonate, requiring significant steroid synthesis to maintain electrolyte balance. Thus the reference ranges for renin and aldosterone in the first 3 months of life are significantly higher than at any other time. As a result, the neonate may produce notable amounts of aldosterone and aldosterone precursor steroids under times of stress and volume depletion. The drive for aldosterone production gradually decreases after birth as expression of the mineralocorticoid receptor increases.

Detectable levels of 17OHP in the serum of normal neonates occurs after birth, but this should fall rapidly within the first few days. These levels may be particularly marked if the infant is premature, but this finding is partly dependent on the specificity of the assay used for analysis as some fetal steroids interfere with immunoassays.

1.2.3 Adolescent Period

After approximately 5 years of age, the ZR begins to form in a process known as adrenarche that may continue to the age of 9–10 years of age. This stage is characterised by an increase in 17,20 lyase activity, primarily related to increased cytochrome b5 expression, and ultimately results in the production of adrenal androgen, particularly DHEA. This process influences the development of secondary sexual characteristics, particularly the development of pubic hair and altered sweat composition and adult body odour. This is particularly apparent in females where adrenal androgens drive most of the early androgenic changes of puberty. In males the process may be indistinguishable from early testicular androgen (testosterone) effects that occur at the start of gonadal puberty (pubarche).

With ageing, DHEA and DHEAS decline to 10–20% of levels seen in young adults, the result of decreased production.

1.3 Steroid Metabolism and Excretion

The synthesis of adrenal steroids may be thought of as only the first half of the steroid story. After synthesis, steroids undergo a complex process of peripheral metabolism and eventual excretion (Fig. 1.11). It is ultimately the occurrence and context of the steroid metabolites that allow for the diagnosis of disorders of steroidogenesis rather than the free steroid hormone itself. The metabolism of steroids occurs for two reasons, namely, to regulate their peripheral activity and to prepare them for excretion by increasing their water solubility.

Peripheral hormone actions are largely regulated by local activation and deactivation at the sites of interest. The foremost mechanism for altering the activity of the circulating hormones is via oxidation and reduction of the steroid structures. A key example of one such reaction is the conversion of cortisol (active hormone) to cortisone (inactive hormone) via oxidation or reduction of the 11-oxy group by the enzyme 11β-hydroxysteroid dehydrogenase (11βHSD).

Most of the enzymatic steps involved in preparing a steroid for excretion take place in the liver and involve the reduction of the Δ4-double bond as well as the interconversion of hydroxyl and oxo groups on the periphery of the steroid molecule (C3, C17 and C20) or at its middle (C11). The steroid hormones are also subject to hepatic phase I and phase II metabolism, by conjugation to glucuronate or sulphate.

1.3.1 Reduction of the Δ4 Bond (C5)

Reduction of the Δ4 bond within the steroid structure occurs mainly via the actions of 5α- and 5β-reductase. This process occurs within the liver catalysed by the 5α-reductase 1 isoform that is mainly responsible for the steroid catabolism but also by 5α-reductase 2, an enzyme found mainly in male reproductive tissue that is responsible for testosterone activation to dihydrotestosterone (DHT). Both isoforms have been identified in the liver of neonates and adults, and it is thought that the type 2 isoform is principally involved in the catabolism of C21 steroids, while the type 1 isoform largely contributes to the catabolism of C19 steroids. Neither isoform has been demonstrated in fetal livers between weeks 13 and 19, with weak activity only present for the type 1 isoform at about 20–24 weeks of gestations. There is only one 5β-reductase, the aldo-keto reductase AKR1D1, expressed in the liver; therefore its activity is affected by conditions such as cholestasis, hepatitis, liver failure and early life (i.e., immature liver enzymes in the neonatal period) leading to a reduction in 5β-reduced steroids and a resulting predominance of 5α-reduced metabolites as is evident in the neonatal urine steroid profile. The importance of 5α-reductase in human development is discussed in Chap. 11.

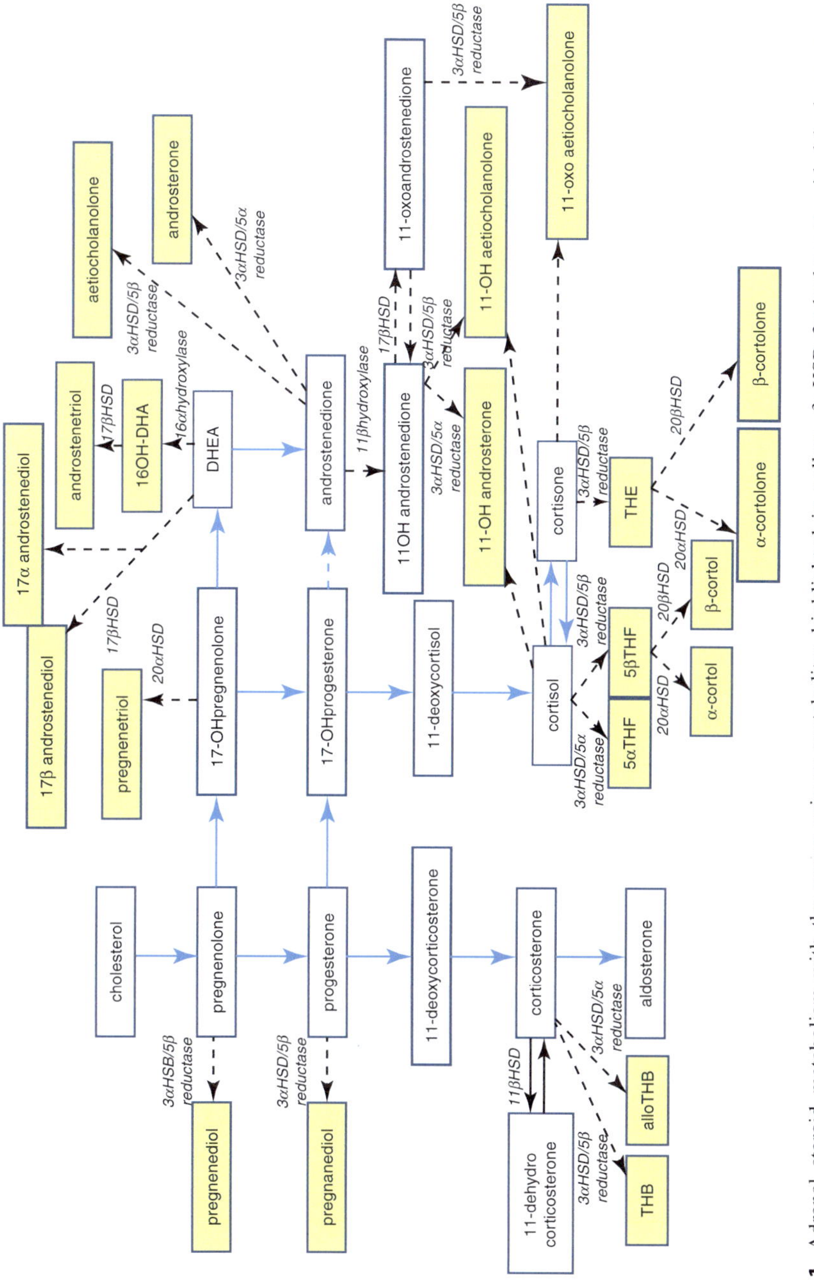

Fig. 1.11 Adrenal steroid metabolism with the major urinary metabolites highlighted in yellow. *3αHSD* 3α-hydroxysteroid dehydrogenase, *11βHSD* 11β-hydroxysteroid dehydrogenase, *20βHSD* 20β-hydroxysteroid dehydrogenase, *20αHSD* 20α-hydroxysteroid dehydrogenase, *17βHSD* 17β-hydroxysteroid dehydrogenase

1.3.2 Oxidation and Reduction of the Steroid Terminals

Oxidation or reduction of the hydroxyls on carbons C3, C17 and C20 of the Δ^4-3-keto steroids plays a central role both in hormone activity regulation and metabolism and excretion. The aldo-keto reductase (AKR1C) family of enzymes can act as 3-, 17- and 20-keto steroid reductases forming 3α/β, 17β and 20-hydroxymetabolites. AKR1C3 is a peripheral enzyme that catalyses the formation of 17β-hydroxylated from 17-oxo steroids, while AKR1C1 is primarily a 20-keto steroid reductase. While these reactions may proceed in both directions, in practice the reactions proceed in a preferential direction depending on local subcellular cofactor availability. It is also clear that although these reactions may favour a particular steroid position, they may also catalyse the oxidoreduction of other steroid locations and work with a variety of substrates. This may be a source of some confusion, since the names given to these enzymes often reflect the order of their discovery, rather than their preferred reaction affinity. Expression of AKR1C3 in the fetal adrenal has been associated with the ACTH-dependent increase in fetal testosterone production.

It is thought that AKR1C1, acting in conjunction with 5β-reductase (AKR1D1), forms the major route for steroid catabolism in the adult liver, with ARK1C4 (also known as 3α-hydroxysteroid dehydrogenase type 1) the major enzyme catalysing 3α-oxidation.

Other enzymes from the 17β-hydroxysteroid dehydrogenase family are also able to dehydrogenate the hydroxyl group at C17. As discussed further in Chap. 10, one of these, 17βHSD3, is a cause of a male disorder of sex differentiation.

1.3.3 Oxidation and Reduction of the Steroid Centre

The major enzyme responsible for the metabolism of mid-steroid oxo group at C11 is 11βHSD. There are two isoforms acting either as a reductase (11βHSD1) or an oxidase (11βHSD2). 11βHSD1 is found predominantly in the liver and subcutaneous fat and serves to regulate the actions of cortisol in these glucocorticoid responsive tissues. 11βHSD2 is found mainly in the kidney and colon and plays a key role in minimising the mineralocorticoid action of cortisol in these tissues. This process is discussed in more detail in the context of 11βHSD deficiency in Chap. 12. 11βHSD2 activity is high immediately after birth resulting in rapid conversion of cortisol to cortisone, thus tetrahydrocortisone (THE), and particularly the 6-hydroxylated form of THE is the predominant neonatal metabolite and not tetrahydrocortisol.

1.3.4 Hydroxylation of Steroids

Hydroxylation of steroids is a key feature of their metabolism, particularly in the perinatal period. This process is performed by the P450 enzyme family described earlier. The main P450 enzymes involved with the metabolism and excretion of steroids are the CYP2 and CYP3 enzymes. The actions and resulting steroid metabolites produced by the CYP enzymes are detailed in each chapter in reference to the specific normal or disease scenarios.

The CYP3A family of enzymes, particularly CYP3A7, is responsible for up to 50% of CYP activity in the fetus and neonate and for the 16α-hydroxylation of steroids such as DHEA. The enzyme plays only a minor role in adult steroid metabolism. After about the first week of life, CYP3A4 and then CYP3A5 expression begins to increase. CYP3A4 has the ability to add 6β-hydroxyl groups on to the steroid molecule, a situation that is particularly apparent following induction of the enzyme with certain drug treatments when the output of 6β-hydroxycortisol is significantly increased.

The CYP2C family of enzymes are poorly expressed in fetal tissue and only increase in expression shortly after birth until adulthood where they represent major routes for steroid metabolism. In particular, the CYP2C9 and CYP2C19 enzymes predominate.

1.3.5 Conjugation of Steroids

Following the initial oxidation, reduction and hydroxylation of steroids described above, the final steps in metabolism before excretion involve their conjugation to large polar molecules, either glucuronate or sulphate. This process is catalysed by either UDP-glucuronyltransferases (UGTs) or sulphotransferases (SULT), respectively. During the fetal and neonatal periods, very little UGT activity is demonstrated, with the majority of metabolites excreted as sulphate conjugates. This process is covered in more detail in the sulphotransferase Chap. 13. The transferase enzyme SULT2A1 is not seen in the neocortex at any fetal stage but is in the transitional zone and highest in the fetal zone cells. After the post-natal involution of the fetal zone, SULT2A1 activity is relatively low until the development of the ZR preceding adrenarche.

Further Reading

Miller WL, Auchus RJ. The molecular biology, biochemistry, and physiology of human steroidogenesis and its disorders. Endocr Rev. 2011;32:81–151.

Shackleton CHL, Honour JW, Taylor NF. Metabolism of fetal and neonatal adrenal steroids. J Steroid Biochem. 1979;11:523–9.

Strauss Jerome F, I II, Martinez F, Kiriakidou M. Placental steroid hormone synthesis: unique features and unanswered questions. Biol Reprod. 1996;54:303–11.

Moss GP. The nomenclature of steroids: recommendations by the IUPAC–IUB joint commission on biochemical nomenclature. Eur J Biochem. 1989;186:429–58.

2 Overview of Adrenocortical Pathophysiology

Oliver Clifford-Mobley

2.1 Introduction

The adrenal glands are a pair of endocrine organs, which sit above the kidneys. In healthy adults they are 4–6 g in mass; the right gland is pyramidal in shape and the left more crescent shaped. Each adrenal gland comprises two embryologically distinct sections: an outer cortex and inner medulla. The adrenal cortex is derived from mesodermal anlagen and is one of the two principal sites of steroid hormone synthesis in the body, along with the gonads. The adrenal medulla is derived from the embryonic neural crest and is the principal site of catecholamine (adrenaline and noradrenaline) synthesis in the body. The cortex and medulla are enclosed within the adrenal capsule, and the whole gland lies within the renal fascia. These two sections of the adrenal function largely independently, and the remainder of this chapter will focus on the adrenal cortex alone.

The adult adrenal cortex comprises three layers, and, although the steroid hormones share a common biosynthetic pathway, each layer is the site of synthesis for a different steroid end product. The relative sizes of the three layers therefore match the relative amounts of the hormones required for normal physiology. The principal mineralocorticoid, aldosterone, is synthesised in the zona glomerulosa (~15% of the cortex); the principal glucocorticoid, cortisol, is synthesised in the zona fasciculata (~75%); the adrenal androgens are synthesised in the zona reticularis (~10%).

There is also a fetal adrenal zone that lies at the boundary between the cortex and medulla. This makes up the majority of the adrenal cortex at birth and

O. Clifford-Mobley
Department of Clinical Biochemistry, University Hospitals Bristol NHS Foundation Trust, Bristol, UK
e-mail: oliver.clifford-mobley@nhs.net

G. Rumsby, G. M. Woodward (eds.), *Disorders of Steroidogenesis*,
https://doi.org/10.1007/978-3-319-96364-8_2

slowly involutes over the first 18 months of life to leave the adult zona glomerulosa and fasciculata, though the zona reticularis remains indistinct until around 5 years of age. The balance of steroid hormones produced by the fetal adrenal is slightly different compared to the adult adrenal. The fetal adrenal zone does not express much 3β-hydroxysteroid dehydrogenase (3βHSD), which manifests in a greater synthesis of Δ5 steroids, for example, dehydroepiandrosterone (DHEA) and DHEA sulphate (DHEAS). The fetal adrenal is able to synthesise cortisol from approximately 8 weeks of gestation, but this is rapidly metabolised by 11β-hydroxysteroid dehydrogenase type 2 (11βHSD2) to cortisone, which is the 11-oxo equivalent of cortisol. Aldosterone synthesis can be much higher, which manifests in a much higher upper limit of normal for this steroid in the neonatal period.

2.2 Steroids and Their Homeostasis

The three principal adrenal steroid hormones have different primary functions and therefore different homeostatic control mechanisms. There is however some overlap in both activity, particularly with the intermediates, and regulation, for example by ACTH. It is possible to have a pathology that selectively affects one or more of the hormones, as well as pathologies that affect the entire adrenal cortex. An understanding of the different regulatory pathways is useful to explain the clinical features of adrenocortical disease.

2.2.1 Aldosterone

The function of mineralocorticoids is to promote sodium, and hence fluid, retention in the renal tubule. Adequate mineralocorticoid reserve is essential for maintaining the circulating volume, particularly in the neonatal period.

A drop in pressure at the efferent arteriole of the glomerulus, or in the concentration of sodium in tubular fluid, is the stimulus for release of renin from the juxtaglomerular apparatus. Renin is a proteolytic enzyme which cleaves angiotensinogen in the circulation to angiotensin I, which is in turn cleaved by angiotensin-converting enzyme to angiotensin II, an octapeptide. Angiotensin II acts on the adrenal to stimulate synthesis of aldosterone which acts on the mineralocorticoid receptors (MR) of the collecting duct to promote sodium retention (at the expense of potassium and/or hydrogen ion). This regulatory pathway is termed the renin–angiotensin–aldosterone system (RAAS).

In normal health the RAAS maintains healthy blood pressure. It is worth noting that the amount of salt in the modern Western diet is high enough such that sodium retention is not normally critical. However, in acute illness with diarrhoea and/or vomiting, adequate aldosterone production is vital to maintain the circulating volume.

2.2.2 Cortisol

Glucocorticoids are important counterregulatory hormones (i.e. act to increase glucose synthesis and release into the circulation), and an increased cortisol is part of the normal response to stress. Glucocorticoids also have a role in regulating the immune system. Cortisol also has mineralocorticoid properties but is inactivated by 11βHSD2 in the kidney to prevent it stimulating the MR.

The driver for cortisol synthesis is adrenocorticotropic hormone (ACTH), a peptide hormone secreted by the anterior pituitary. The secretion of ACTH is itself under the control of corticotropin-releasing hormone (CRH) secreted by the hypothalamus. Cortisol exerts negative feedback at the hypothalamus to maintain normal homeostasis. This regulatory pathway is termed the hypothalamus–pituitary–adrenal (HPA) axis.

Correct functioning of the HPA axis is required for the body to mount the physiological response to stress. It also has a strong diurnal rhythm with a peak of cortisol production occurring in early morning, which is associated with waking from sleep.

2.2.3 Adrenal Androgens

Adrenal androgens are the principal source of androgenic function in females, but are not significant in men due to the greater androgenic activity of testosterone produced by the gonads. It is not thought that adrenal androgens are essential for life in the adult. However, although the mechanism is not fully understood, they are involved in triggering puberty.

Adrenal androgens (DHEA(S), androstenedione (A4), androstenediol) have little androgenic activity compared to testosterone. They do however provide a large circulating pool of androgens which can be converted to testosterone (and thence to oestradiol, E2) in the periphery by 17β-hydroxysteroid dehydrogenase. In the male the contribution of the adrenal to total testosterone is very low (~1%); however in the female up to half of the circulating testosterone is ultimately derived from adrenal androgens. In common with cortisol, ACTH functions as a stimulator of adrenal androgen synthesis, though the adrenal androgens do not exhibit the same negative feedback on pituitary ACTH production as does cortisol. The presence of another regulatory pathway is also suggested by the phenomenon of adrenarche, which occurs independently of ACTH. However, the identity of a specific adrenal androgen-stimulating hormone has not been confirmed. Adrenarche occurs from around 5 years of age, as a result of the expansion of the zona reticularis and increased expression of cytochrome b5 that promotes 17,20 lyase activity of the 17α-hydroxylase enzyme resulting in increased synthesis of adrenal androgens, in particular DHEAS. It leads to appearance of pubic hair but not other secondary sex characteristics. The growth of the zona reticularis lasts until post-puberty when the full adult adrenal size is reached. By this time the gonads have taken over as the predominant source of sex steroids.

2.2.4 Exogenous Steroids

Steroid hormone replacement therapy is required for patients with hypofunctioning adrenals, of whatever aetiology. This usually takes the form of steroids with glucocorticoid activity (e.g. hydrocortisone), mineralocorticoid activity (e.g. fludrocortisone) or both (e.g. prednisolone). Supplementation with DHEA is only recommended in those patients with low libido, depressive symptoms and low energy levels who are otherwise optimally controlled with glucocorticoid and mineralocorticoids.

Replacement steroids can include compounds chemically identical to the endogenous hormones (e.g. hydrocortisone) and also synthetic compounds. The latter group is large and expanding and presents a challenge to the interpretation of laboratory steroid measurement. The common immunoassay-based methods for most of the major serum steroids have variable cross-reactivity with synthetic steroids. A urine steroid profile (USP) analysed by mass spectrometry has the advantage of being able to distinguish endogenous from synthetic steroids. However, in clinical practice, the quantitation of synthetic steroids is rarely undertaken.

2.3 Types of Pathology

In general it is possible to divide adrenocortical pathology into the inborn errors of steroidogenesis and acquired pathologies, which are dealt with separately in the remainder of this book. Urine steroid profiling is a very versatile analytical method which can help to make the diagnosis for all of the former and can be informative in many of the latter. Notable exceptions include gonadal steroid disorders, for example, aromatase deficiency and androgen receptor defects, where no useful urinary markers are present. Even so, the USP may be helpful even in these cases to exclude other overlapping disorders of sex development. The clinical features of adrenocortical disease are determined in general by deficiency or excess of the various steroid hormone products. Therefore, a discussion of adrenocortical pathology follows logically on from a division into the deficiency and excess of glucocorticoids, mineralocorticoids and adrenal androgens. The effect on each class of steroid hormone due to the inborn errors presented in this book is summarised in Table 2.1.

2.3.1 Adrenal Deficiency States

2.3.1.1 Congenital Adrenal Hyperplasia

The inborn errors of metabolism which result in ineffectual cortisol biosynthesis are termed the congenital adrenal hyperplasias (CAH), of which there are five types. By the far the most common (~90% of cases) is 21-hydroxylase (CYP21) deficiency

Table 2.1 Effect of inborn errors on each class of steroid hormone

Disorder	Effect on glucocorticoids	Effect on mineralocorticoids	Effect on sex steroids	Chapters
21-Hydroxylase	Hypocortisolism	Salt-losing	Virilising	4
11β-Hydroxylase	Hypocortisolism	Hypertensive	Virilising	5
3β-Hydroxysteroid dehydrogenase	Hypocortisolism	Salt-losing	Virilising	6
17α-Hydroxylase	Hypocortisolism	Hypertensive	M: 46,XY DSD F: 1° infertility	7
Lipoid CAH and cholesterol 20–22 lyase	Hypocortisolism	Salt-losing	M: 46,XY DSD F: 1° infertility	8
Aldosterone synthase	None	Salt-losing	None	9
Glucocorticoid remedial hyperaldosteronism	None	Hypertensive	None	5
17β-Hydroxysteroid dehydrogenase	None	None	M: 46,XY DSD F: none	10
5α-Reductase	None	None	M: 46,XY DSD F: none	11
11β-Hydroxysteroid dehydrogenase type 2	Hypercortisolism	Hypertensive	None	12
Steroid sulfatase	None	None	None	13
P450 Oxidoreductase	Hypocortisolism	None/salt losing	M: 46,XY DSD F: virilising in utero	14
Smith Lemli Opitz	Hypocortisolism (rarely)	Salt-losing (rarely)	M: 46,XY DSD F: none	14
Adrenoleukodystrophy	Hypocortisolism	Salt-losing	None	17

(see Chap. 4). 11β-Hydroxylase (CYP11; see Chap. 5), 17α-hydroxylase (CYP17, see Chap. 7) and 3βHSD (see Chap. 6) deficiencies affect other enzymes involved in the cortisol biosynthetic pathway. Lipoid CAH is due to deficiency of steroid acute regulatory protein (StAR), which, along with cholesterol side-chain cleavage (P450scc), occurs right at the start of the steroid pathway and hence affects all other steroid hormones (see Chap. 8). All forms of CAH are similar in that they cause hypocortisolism but with key differences due to the effects on other parts of the adrenal steroid biosynthetic pathway. Because many of the enzymes involved in steroid biosynthesis are common to more than one pathway, some forms of CAH result in reduced synthesis of mineralocorticoids and/or adrenal androgens. In addition hypocortisolism itself releases negative feedback in the HPA axis and leads to increased stimulation of the adrenal by ACTH, which causes the hyperplasia. This in turn can drive increased synthesis of further steroid hormones due to their common metabolic routes. Therefore, although CAH is an inborn error of metabolism which causes a loss of function change in cortisol biosynthesis, it can paradoxically lead to adrenal hyperfunction in other steroid pathways.

It is possible to divide CAH into the virilising (CYP21, CYP11, 3βHSD) and non-virilising (CYP17, lipoid CAH) forms. In the former case, synthesis of adrenal androgens is not impaired by the specific metabolic block. The increased ACTH drive to the adrenal engendered by hypocortisolism therefore causes an 'overflow' down the androgen biosynthetic pathway. In non-virilising CAH, the metabolic block also renders adrenal androgen synthesis ineffectual; therefore no hyperandrogenism occurs.

Another division is between the salt-losing (CYP21, 3βHSD, lipoid CAH) and hypertensive (CYP11, CYP17) forms of CAH. In the former case, there is ineffectual mineralocorticoid synthesis. In the hypertensive CAH, the metabolic block does not preclude mineralocorticoid biosynthesis. The increased ACTH drive therefore causes unregulated oversynthesis of mineralocorticoids; however this is not in the form of aldosterone itself but rather 11-deoxycorticosterone (DOC) which has slightly weaker mineralocorticoid activity. Because of the normal physiological response of the RAAS to hypertension, aldosterone production may be actually suppressed in these cases.

2.3.1.2 Other Inherited Adrenal Diseases

An inborn error of metabolism specifically affecting aldosterone synthesis also exists (see Chap. 9). The deficient enzyme, aldosterone synthase, catalyses the final steps in the biosynthesis of aldosterone, and it is only found in the zona glomerulosa. Therefore, cortisol and adrenal androgen production is unaffected, and symptoms relate to salt loss and hypovolaemia.

Both CYP21 and CYP17 rely on cytochrome P450 oxidoreductase (POR) for electron transfer. Therefore deficiency of POR causes a mixed 21- and 17-hydroxylase deficiency (see Chap. 14).

2.3.1.3 Pan-Adrenal Hypofunction

Pan-adrenal hypofunction is usually due to acquired adrenal disease unrelated to steroid synthesis per se (see Chap. 17). Adrenal hypofunction unrelated to an inborn error is characterised by deficiency of all steroid hormone products. The common causes are infective (e.g. granulomatous disease, HIV) and autoimmune (Addison's disease). The onset is often insidious but if unchecked can lead to an adrenal crisis. A characteristic feature of primary adrenal insufficiency is hyperpigmentation of the skin due to the increased pituitary production of ACTH, which is no longer subject to normal negative feedback. The pituitary synthesis of ACTH produces melanocyte-stimulating hormone in an equimolar amount, the latter hormone promoting the hyperpigmentation.

The steroidogenic factor 1 (SF1) regulates many genes involved in steroidogenesis, and mutations in *NR5A1* (the gene encoding SF1) can cause primary adrenal failure and a 46,XY disorder of sexual differentiation.

2.3.2 Pathologies of Adrenal Steroid Hormone Excess

There are two mechanisms by which excessive secretion of one or more of the adrenal steroids may occur: either due to increased stimulation by an upstream factor (secondary) or due to autonomous production (primary). The clinical features will depend on whether there is excessive glucocorticoid, mineralocorticoid or adrenal androgen secretion.

2.3.2.1 Glucocorticoid Excess

Glucocorticoid excess is termed Cushing's syndrome (see Chap. 16) and comprises three distinct disease states, depending on which part of the HPA axis is impaired.

Loss of negative feedback in the HPA axis is the cause of the hypercortisolism of Cushing's disease. The primary pathology in the great majority of cases is an ACTH-secreting tumour in the pituitary. Very rarely there is ectopic ACTH secretion by a different tumour, typically a small cell lung cancer. As a consequence of the increased ACTH drive, there is a bilateral adrenal hyperplasia and a characteristic loss of the normal diurnal rhythm of cortisol secretion. Hypercortisolism can also be primary, that is, due to a cortisol-secreting adrenal tumour. In these cases negative feedback in the HPA axis reduces ACTH secretion, and there is suppression of the contralateral adrenal.

The clinical symptoms are similar irrespective of the aetiology and develop as a result of hypercortisolism: obesity, hypertension, pro-diabetic state, acne, proximal myopathy and easy bruising.

2.3.2.2 Mineralocorticoid Excess

Increased mineralocorticoid activity causes enhanced sodium and water retention in the distal renal tubule and consequent hypertension that is characteristically associated with hypokalaemia and metabolic alkalosis.

Primary aldosteronism (PA), also known as Conn syndrome, arises due to autonomous secretion of aldosterone. This can be from an adrenal adenoma, bilateral adrenal hyperplasia or very rarely due to glucocorticoid remedial aldosteronism (GRA). The aetiology of GRA is a genetic variant in which the promoter region for *CYP11B1* (the gene encoding CYP11, the last step in cortisol biosynthesis) is fused to *CYP11B2* (the gene encoding aldosterone synthase). This results in aldosterone production coming under the direct influence of ACTH levels rather than the RAAS (see Chap. 5).

Several other pathological states mimic primary aldosteronism, but with low aldosterone production, and the mineralocorticoid activity coming from other adrenal steroids. As already mentioned, Cushing's syndrome gives rise to hypertension. The mechanism is that the increased cortisol overwhelms the capacity of renal 11βHSD2, and therefore unregulated stimulation of the MR by cortisol occurs.

Reduced activity of 11βHSD2 itself has the same effect, even in the presence of normal cortisol. This is termed apparent mineralocorticoid excess (AME) and is either an inborn error of metabolism or acquired due to inhibition of the 11βHSD2, for example, by glycyrrhizic acid (in liquorice). In the two hypertensive forms of CAH, CYP11 and CYP17, the excess mineralocorticoid is DOC.

The pseudohyperaldosteronisms (PHA) are inborn errors affecting the RAAS in which there is no actual mineralocorticoid excess but rather their unregulated action on the distal tubule. In PHA type 1 (Liddle syndrome), there is a gain of function mutation in the epithelial sodium channel (ENaC). In PHA type 2, there is gain of function mutation in the MR.

Mineralocorticoid excess secondary to elevated renin occurs in renovascular hypertension, which is due to renal artery stenosis. More rarely there are inborn errors of renal tubule function that cause fluid loss and consequent overactivation of the RAAS—Bartter and Gitelman syndromes-however in these cases, there is hypotension.

2.3.2.3 Adrenal Androgen Excess

As already discussed above, CAH causes an increased ACTH drive, and, although these diseases are adrenal deficiency states, the virilising forms often manifest as adrenal androgen excess. There is a so-called simple virilising form of 21-hydroxylase deficiency. In these cases the metabolic block is not complete, and the patient is able to produce adequate cortisol reserves but at the expense of excessive ACTH stimulation. The presenting features are therefore solely related to the androgen excess. In other virilising forms of CAH, the presenting features usually include hypocortisolism as well.

More rarely an adrenal tumour can present as an isolated hyperandrogenic state (hirsutism, virilisation, acne, deepening of the voice). This is due to autonomous production of adrenal androgens, principally DHEA, and independently of ACTH stimulation.

2.3.2.4 Adrenal Adenoma, Incidentaloma and Adrenocortical Carcinoma

Adrenal tumours can be functional and non-functional, as well as benign or malignant (see Chap. 15). A benign functional adrenal adenoma typically produces just one of the steroid hormones in excess, cortisol (adrenal Cushing's), aldosterone (Conn's) or DHEA. A malignant adrenocortical carcinoma is characterised by hypersecretion of both cortisol and androgens, as well as other intermediate steroids. The presence of abnormal steroid metabolites in urine can be used to aid characterisation of the tumour type and monitor treatment.

With the increased use of sensitive imaging techniques, the phenomenon of the adrenal incidentaloma has become relatively common in the setting of secondary care. An adrenal incidentaloma is defined as an adrenal mass detected on imaging not performed for suspected adrenal disease (e.g. for investigation of abdominal or back pain). In contrast with other adrenal pathologies where specific investigations are indicated by the presenting symptoms, with incidentaloma a broad spectrum of testing may need to be employed in order to rule out a functional adenoma. The results of imaging investigations are also useful in this regard because functional adenomata are typically lipid rich (cholesterol being the substrate for steroid hormone synthesis) and hence have a typical appearance on imaging.

Further Reading

Adrenal Pathophysiology

Miller WL, Auchus RJ. The molecular biology, biochemistry, and physiology of human steroidogenesis and its disorders. Endocr Rev. 2011;32(1):81–151.

Steroid Profiling: Analytical Perspectives

3

Gary M. Woodward and Gill Rumsby

3.1 Introduction

Steroid analysis may be performed using many different analytical techniques, ranging from radioimmunoassay and electrophoresis to GC and LC–MS/MS. Steroids may also be measured in a range of biological fluids including blood, urine and saliva. It was not until the 1960s that the concept of multicomponent steroid analysis was first mentioned. The combined analysis of steroid metabolites in urine (urine steroid profile) has long been useful for the diagnosis of disorders of steroidogenesis and adrenal disease, with the most prominent utility in our Institute's experience being the investigation of ambiguous genitalia, precocious puberty/premature adrenarche, Cushing's syndrome, tumours, hyperandrogenism, hypertension, problems of growth and development, renal salt loss and male and female disorders of sex development (DSD).

It was probably in the mid-1960s that the term 'steroid profile' was first adopted. While many definitions of this term might apply, they all encompass the notion that multiple components are used as a diagnostic test and typically provide information beyond just the numerical values for each discrete component. This is exemplified by the fact that some of the most important steroid species may be present in the lowest abundance, setting steroid profiling aside from most other diagnostic profiles. Ultimately, the goal of the steroid profile is to produce a single snapshot of all components of interest, determined in a non-discriminatory manner that in the presence of clinical context can delineate disease from normal states.

Notable steroids in human physiology and pathophysiology may be separated into several distinct groups: primary steroid hormones, secondary steroid hormones,

G. M. Woodward (✉) · G. Rumsby
Department of Clinical Biochemistry, University College London Hospitals, London, UK
e-mail: Gary.Woodward1@nhs.net

G. Rumsby, G. M. Woodward (eds.), *Disorders of Steroidogenesis*,
https://doi.org/10.1007/978-3-319-96364-8_3

steroid precursors and terminal steroid metabolites. Primary steroid hormones represent those with biological endocrine function. Secondary steroids usually proximate the primary steroids in the biosynthetic pathway, while terminal metabolites are excreted in the urine or bile as either free steroids or as conjugates with sulphate or glucuronide.

Although steroid analysis is performed on most biological fluids, urine steroid analysis is preferred over plasma in the context of investigating disorders of steroidogenesis for three key reasons: firstly it is non-invasive (particularly useful in neonatal cases); secondly it is non-selective, giving an overall view of steroidogenesis; and, thirdly, an approximation of total 24-h steroid production can be made from a random sample. Urine steroid profiling (USP) has progressed significantly over the past decades, moving from gas chromatography (GC) to GC/mass spectrometry (GC/MS) GC/MS and liquid chromatography/MS (LC–MS/MS). Immunoassays and similar methodologies have also been widely used for quantification of steroid hormones in routine diagnostics. Although alternative steroid profiling methodologies are available, GC/MS has predominated as the favoured technique for more than 40 years; its strength rests with its versatility.

LC–MS/MS is inarguably the primary method for serum steroid hormone analysis in most clinical laboratories and for good reason. It requires small sample volumes and has a high degree of specificity and short analysis times. Much of the drive for a move to LC–MS/MS analysis has been due to issues with steroid specificity by other routine techniques such as immunoassays. Indeed LC–MS/MS analysis of steroids is widely accepted as the gold standard for the quantification of individual steroids using the separation of reference steroids. To do this, analytical procedures need to be tailored to the target analyte/analytes which intrinsically requires a decision to be made in advance to measure a specific group of compounds. However, LC–MS/MS is limited in its ability to define novel and varied metabolomes. GC/MS, while unsuited to rapid high-sensitivity analysis of specific compounds, remains the most powerful tool for assessing the steroid metabolome. While metabolomic LC–MS/MS methods have advanced greatly over the decades, currently the techniques and expertise required remain beyond the scope of most current clinical laboratories. The ability to measure a large range of steroid metabolites remains particularly accessible to urine steroid analysis by GC/MS.

The following chapter aims to provide the reader with a basic technical understanding of urine steroid profiling by GC/MS, to describe the influence of physiology on the 'normal' profile and provide an awareness of some important pitfalls and diagnostic caveats.

3.2 Isolation of the Steroids

Historically the extraction of unconjugated steroids has favoured the use of solvent partitioning with solvents such as methylene chloride or diethyl ether. However solid-phase extraction (SPE) has long been the standard approach for the extraction of steroid conjugates from aqueous solutions such as urine. SPE is a sample preparation technique that uses solid particle chromatographic packing material, usually contained in a cartridge-type device, to chemically separate the different components of a sample. Samples are nearly always in the liquid state. Solid packing materials such as Amberlite XAD-2 resin have been used to retain the conjugated steroids during SPE, although C18 cartridges (Sep-Pak) predominate today with the development of bonded-phase silica supports for high-performance liquid chromatography. The solid packing material absorbs the steroid conjugate in a water-based solution (i.e. urine or plasma) onto its surface for later recovery by elution with a polar solvent such as ethanol. The eluted steroid conjugates may then be further prepared for chromatographic analysis.

It can be helpful to separate some steroid species to make the interpretation somewhat simpler. This situation particularly applies to the analysis of neonatal steroids that are excreted as highly sulphated conjugates. This is achieved by the pre-isolation of mono- and disulphates using Sephadex LH-20 and a saline-saturated methanol–chloroform solvent mixture. Free steroid and glucuronide conjugates are not retained by the column, while mono- and disulphated steroid conjugates can be eluted with ethanol. This method remains the most widely adopted means for grouping steroid sulphate fractions.

3.3 Hydrolysis of Conjugates

Following steroid isolation and prior to analytical analyses, the conjugated steroid species require liberation to form free steroids. This is typically achieved by enzymatic hydrolysis, although other methods such as acid hydrolysis have been used. Quantitative hydrolysis of all urinary steroids can be difficult to achieve owning to the large variability in enzyme preparations and stability. Enzyme hydrolysis is typically achieved using β-glucuronidase usually found as purified bacterial (*Escherichia coli*) preparations, digestive juices of the Roman snail (*Helix pomatia*), limpet (*Patella vulgata*) homogenates or bovine liver homogenates. It should be noted that most β-glucuronidase preparations also possess varying degrees of sulphatase activity, *Helix pomatia* isolates being particularly useful in this regard. These tend to be very crude preparations and have considerable batch-to-batch variation warranting validation prior to use. Advances in enzyme expression and engineering have improved consistency and yield but at a price.

The enzymatic hydrolysis of steroids represents a significant methodological bottleneck for urine steroid profiling. Significant amounts of work have gone into optimising the hydrolysis of conjugated urine steroids with the summary outcome being that temperature has little effect on the hydrolysis of most steroids with some notable exceptions. The hydrolysis of dehydroepiandrosterone sulphate (DHEAS) is improved at higher temperatures while the recovery of both androsterone and aetiocholanolone falls. The optimal temperature for hydrolysis is between 52 and 60 °C, depending on the enzyme preparation used. It is clear that longer hydrolysis times produce greater yields and incubation times of 3 h at the higher temperature or overnight at a lower temperature of 37 °C are commonly used. The yield of 5α-reduced steroids, particularly those with an 11-hydroxyl group, for example, 5α-tetrahydrocortisol (5αTHF), can be improved by the inclusion of ascorbate in the hydrolysis reaction. Following hydrolysis, it is favourable to purify the steroid mixture prior to derivatisation. The freed steroids may be recovered by Sep-Pak SPE as previously described.

3.4 Derivatisation

Unlike other methods for steroid profiling, GC/MS has the distinct disadvantage of needing to protect the thermally labile groups from the high temperatures required for volatilisation and separation. Many methods are available for the protection of labile steroid species, although derivatisation (the transformation of a chemical compound into another by altering one or more of its functional groups) with methoxyamine and *N*-trimethylsilylimidazole (MO–TMS derivatives) has become the method of choice, owing to the ease with which carbonyl and hydroxyl groups can be protected (Fig. 3.1). The carbonyl group at carbon 11 that is present in, for example, tetrahydrocortisone (THE), is resistant to methoximation. Following methoximation, the hydroxyls are silylated to trimethylsilyl ethers (TMS). As well as the additional work required to perform derivatisations, this process brings unique challenges relating to the interpretation of urine steroid profiles. Since methyloxime derivatives may be produced in two forms for each carbonyl function (*syn* and *anti* forms), different epimers could be formed for each steroid compound. However, in practice the production of several epimers per steroid is not seen extensively, possibly because they have similar retention times and are not resolved. Some that are clearly resolved include 16α-hydroxyDHEA, 16,18-dihydroxyDHEA and tetrahydrocorticosterone.

Hydroxime (HO) and benzyloxime derivatives (BO-TMS) are also occasionally used to improve separation and identification of some steroid species by shifting their positions on the chromatogram. For example, 17α-hydroxypregnanolone

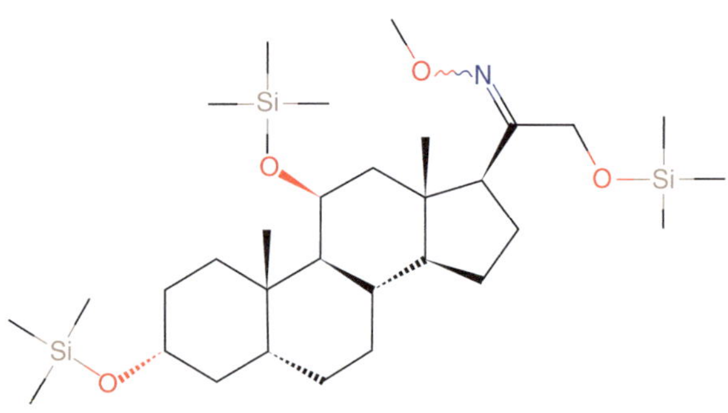

Fig. 3.1 Example of a steroid molecule after derivatisation. The ketone group has been converted to a methyloxime and the hydroxyl groups to trimethylsilyl ethers

co-elutes with 11β-hydroxyandrosterone using MO-TMS derivatization but may be resolved when converted to BO-TMS derivatives.

3.5 Gas Chromatography/Mass Spectrometry (GC/MS)

It was thought that with the advent of tandem MS, GC/MS analysis of steroid would become obsolete. However, while LC–MS/MS of serum steroid hormones dominate the clinical laboratory, the two analytical techniques are complementary rather than competitive.

In simple terms, GC/MS analysis on capillary columns is performed on neutral steroids converted into MO-TMS ethers. GC/MS describes an instrumental technique that comprises two distinct parts, namely, the gas chromatograph (GC) and the mass spectrometer (MS). GC permits the separation of compounds that can be vaporised without decomposition. In brief, a sample solution is injected into the GC system where it is vaporised and moved via a carrier gas (usually helium) onto a chromatographic column. As the analytes flow through the column, they are separated by virtue of their relative interaction with the coating of the column (stationary phase) and the carrier gas (mobile phase). The time at which an analyte elutes from the column (retention time) can be recorded to produce a chromatogram (a plot of analyte elution (retention) as a function of time. When coupled to a MS, the latter part of the column passes through a heated transfer line and ends at the entrance to an ion source (first functional part of the MS) where the analytes eluting from the column are converted to ions. The separated analyte ions are then pulled through a series of quadrupoles producing an oscillating electric field. The analytes pass through the oscillating electric field as a function of their mass and charge to reach a detector (typically an electron multiplier) to produce a mass spectrum (a plot of the ion signal intensity as a function of the mass-to-charge ratio—*m*/*z*). As such, the identification of a steroid is based on its retention time (RT) and its mass spectrum. It is important to state that retention time itself as a means of steroid identification is only relevant to the specific chromatographic system used to determine them. If chromatographic retention data are to be universal or exchangeable between systems and laboratories, they must be independent of the instrument used. As such, the concept of retention index (RI) has been developed. This refers to the retention time of an analyte relative to that of a reference compound. The RI index uses a homologous series of compounds of increasing size. This increase in size is consistent and proportional and involves the sequential addition of methylene groups (known as methylene units—MU) and provides reference points on a scale. The most commonly used system comprises straight-chain saturated hydrocarbons (alkanes). In simple terms, for any given column temperature and stationary phase, the elution times for a series of alkanes are assumed to increase by a given reference value for each additional methylene unit. Where possible, the MUs for each steroid metabolite are provided in each chapter to aid identification.

While most urine steroid profiles are produced in full-scan electron impact mode (non-selective), GC/MS may also be performed in a more selective mode (selected ion monitoring) which enables targeting of low-level compounds that have diagnostic utility, such as metabolites of aldosterone.

Three internal standards (IS), steroid analogues with defined GC/MS characteristics, are used for the identification and quantification of steroids of interest. Common internal standards include 5α-androstane-3α,17α-diol (A), stigmasterol (S) and cholesterol butyrate (CB). A elutes before the naturally occurring steroids, and CB elutes at the end of the chromatogram. S is included as a measure of completeness of the derivatisation, and peak heights for S and CB should be similar. If S is low relative to CB or absent, the derivatisation reaction was poor.

The steroid excretion rates may be calculated from the analyte peak height response relative to the peak height response of a known reference standard at a known concentration. The length of the GC/MS run times required for the profiling of urine steroids means that there is a tendency for the latter eluting steroid peak heights to fall as their peak widths increase. As a result, steroid excretion rates are calculated relative to the A and CB reference standards that elute at the beginning and end of the runs, using a simple regression line calculation relating the fall of the peak height with RT and known IS concentrations. Correction factors may be needed for some steroids that do not meet the ideal peak height, for example, tetrahydrocortisone, possibly related to the instability of the compound as a result of the carbonyl group at C11.

3.6 Urine Steroid Profile (USP) Interpretation

USP are primarily for the investigation of adrenal steroid disorders of steroidogenesis and other adrenal pathologies, gonadal steroid output being too low to contribute much to the profile. An estimate of total cortisol and androgen metabolites can be made as follows:

$$\text{Total cortisol metabolites} = \begin{pmatrix} \text{THE} + \text{THF} + 5\alpha\text{THF} + \alpha\,\text{cortolone} \\ +\beta\,\text{cortolone} + \beta\,\text{cortol} + 11\text{OH androsterone} \end{pmatrix}$$

$$\text{Total androgen metabolites} = \begin{pmatrix} \text{androsterone} + \text{aetiocholanolone} + \text{DHEA} \\ +16\alpha\text{OH DHEA} + \text{androstenetriol} \end{pmatrix}$$

In cases of suspected disorders of steroidogenesis, it is recommended that at least one urine steroid profile is performed, ideally off treatment, to define the disorder and to better inform genetic testing. Urine collections for USP should preferably be 24-h collections in the absence of preservatives if accurate quantitation of cortisol metabolites is required, although random urine samples are perfectly acceptable for the investigation of disorders of steroid metabolism. A short collection may be unavoidable in infants when a diagnosis is not clearly established, and treatment cannot be delayed. Samples should be taken after 3 days of life and ideally after 5 days to avoid interference from maternal and placental steroids. In our experience, assessment of urine creatinine is helpful to ascertain whether the urine is a full 24-h collection or, in the case of a random sample, is particularly dilute or concentrated as this can impact on interpretation. Random samples are also affected by time of day collected. Serum cortisol reaches a peak early in the morning, and it takes at least 2–3 h for free cortisol to be excreted and a further 2 h delay for the metabolites to be synthesised and excreted. Therefore, the output of total cortisol metabolites and androgens is maximal between 12:00 and 15:00. In addition, some of the metabolites themselves have a diurnal rhythm. For example, 5α/5βtetrahydrocortisol (5αTHF/5βTHF) and 20-hydroxy/20-oxo metabolites reach peak levels at approximately 22:00 and trough at approximately 09:00.

GC/MS is typically performed in full-scan electron impact mode for the detection of derivatised steroids. Combining information provided by the chromatography with the mass spectra, a composite picture of the major biosynthetic and catabolic pathways may be formed. A USP chromatogram typically shows peaks for the three internal standards at positions that have been previously established and flanks the peaks of interest. Extracted ion plots may be used for identification and quantification of relevant metabolites. Most peaks on the chromatogram of a normal subject can be attributed to a specific steroid based on its position and relative amount. In general, there are two groups of steroid metabolite peaks on a chromatogram, namely, androgen metabolites and cortisol metabolites. For the most part, androgen metabolites are found at the beginning of the chromatogram, while cortisol metabolites elute later. Intermediate metabolites tend to be found between the androgen and cortisol metabolite groups. For each peak, a mass spectrum (typically in the range 100–800 *m*/*z*) can be obtained. Each mass spectrum represents a 'finger print' for a specific steroid species, providing information on molecular weight and structure (as a function of the *m*/*z* fragment produced from the parent compound). For TMS derivatives of steroids, the molecular ion is often not evident, making interpretation of structure somewhat more difficult. The mass spectrum derives mainly from substitutions in the A and D rings of the steroid and the side chain of the molecule. Most laboratories interpret the mass spectra visually with knowledge of reference mass spectra for commonly occurring steroids (see Appendix A) and with profiles previously obtained in known disorders. This requires some expectation of what the condition is, based both on the clinical information supplied and on prior experience. GC retention times show little variation over time so that direct comparison of archived results with new results is helpful. It is important to remember that the evaluation of the whole USP pattern in relation to clinical context is required for diagnosis and not just individual peaks.

3.7 Changes in the Profile with Age

A representative neonatal profile is given in Fig. 3.2 and a table of common steroids found and their characteristics in Table 3.1. It can be seen that there is a high excretion of 3β-hydroxy-5-ene steroids, for example, 16αOHDHEA and 16-hydroxypregnenolone, in the sulphate fraction reflecting the predominance of

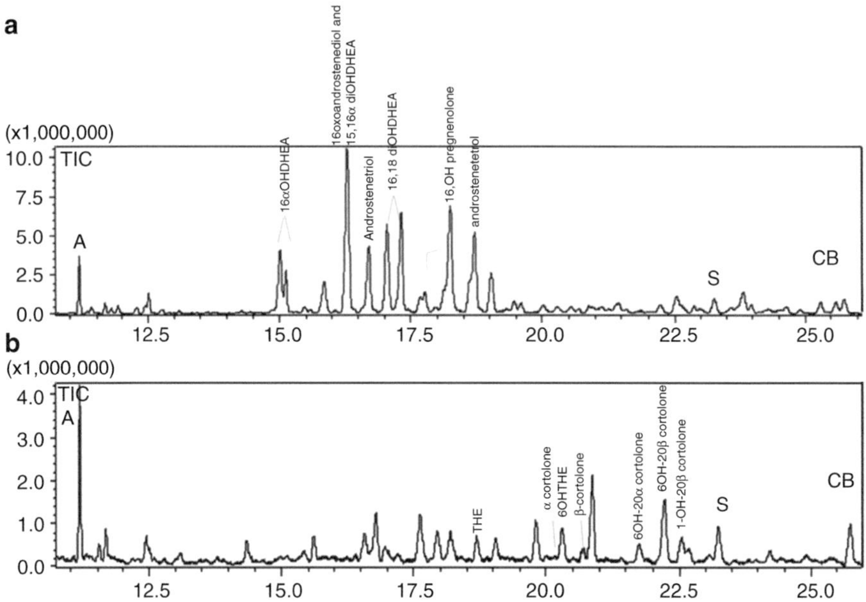

Fig. 3.2 Neonatal urine steroid profile, (a) sulphate fraction, (b) free steroids and glucuronide fraction. Note the predominance of cortisone metabolites in this spectrum compared to Figs. 3.3 and 3.4. A, S and CB denote the internal standards, androstanediol, stigmasterol and cholesterol butyrate, respectively. In this figure and all steroid profiles in this book, the x axis is retention time (minutes). TIC total ion count

Table 3.1 The major steroids found in neonatal urine, retention times (methylene units, MU) of their MO-TMS derivatives and characteristic ions (see appendix for spectra)

Steroid	Trivial name	MU	Ions
Sulphate fraction			
5-Androsten-3β,16α-ol-17-one	16αOH DHEA	27.42	266, 466
5-Androsten-3β,16β-ol-17-one	16βOH DHEA	27.49	266, 466
5-Androsten-3β-ol-16,17-dione and 5-Androsten-3β,15β,16α-triol-17-one	(16-Oxo-androstenediol) and 15,16-dihydroxy-DHEA	28.22	(446, 356) 565, 232
5-Androsten-3β,16α,17β-triol	Androstenetriol	28.47	432, 329
5-Androsten-3β,16a,18-triol-17-one	16,18-Dihydroxy DHEA	28.67	388, 534
5-Pregnen-3α,16α-diol-20-one	16α-Hydroxypregnenolone	29.41	474, 384
5-Androstene-3β,15,16,17-tetrol	Androstenetetrol	29.72	191
0–30 Fraction (free steroids and glucuronides)			
5β-Pregnan-3α,17,21-triol-11,20-dione	THE	29.69	578, 488
5β-Pregnan-3α,17,20α,21-tetrol-11-one	α-Cortolone	30.51	449, 359
5β-Pregnan-3α,6α,17,21-tetrol-11,20-dione	6-Hydroxy-THE	30.80	666, 576
5β-Pregnan-3α,17,20β,21-tetrol-11-one	β-Cortolone	30.82	449, 359
5β-Pregnan-3α,6α,17,20α,21-pentol-11-one	6-Hydroxy-20α-cortolone	31.38	537, 357
5β-Pregnan-3α,6α,17,20β,21-pentol-11-one	6-Hydroxy-20β-cortolone	31.63	537, 357
5β-Pregnan-1,3α,17,20β,21-pentol-11-one	1-Hydroxy-20β-cortolone	31.78	196, 209

fetal adrenal steroids in the neonate. In addition, the major cortisol metabolite is tetrahydrocortisone (THE) and 6-hydroxyTHE rather than THF and 5α-THF illustrating the very active 11βhydroxysteroid dehydrogenase 2 in the neonate and also the predominance of 6α-hydroxylated products at this time. The fetal adrenal metabolites regress over the first month of age but can be present for up to 6 months, particularly if the child is premature, and can be confused with 3β-hydroxysteroid dehydrogenase deficiency, making diagnosis of this disorder difficult early in life (see Chap. 6).

The adult pattern of cortisol metabolites is gradually developed over the first 6 months of life; usually 5α-THF is more dominant than THF at this time, but this gradually settles down to the adult pattern. There is little in the way of adrenal androgen metabolites present prior to adrenarche at age 5–8 years when androsterone and aetiocholanolone become more evident (Fig. 3.3).

In the adult the pattern remains fairly stable over the years although with a decrease in adrenal androgens in later life (Fig. 3.4). The common metabolites in children and adults are given in Table 3.2. It is not uncommon for older males to have an apparent deficiency of 5α-reductase simply through treatment of prostate disorders with 5α-reductase inhibitors finasteride and dutasteride. This pharmacological information is frequently not provided!

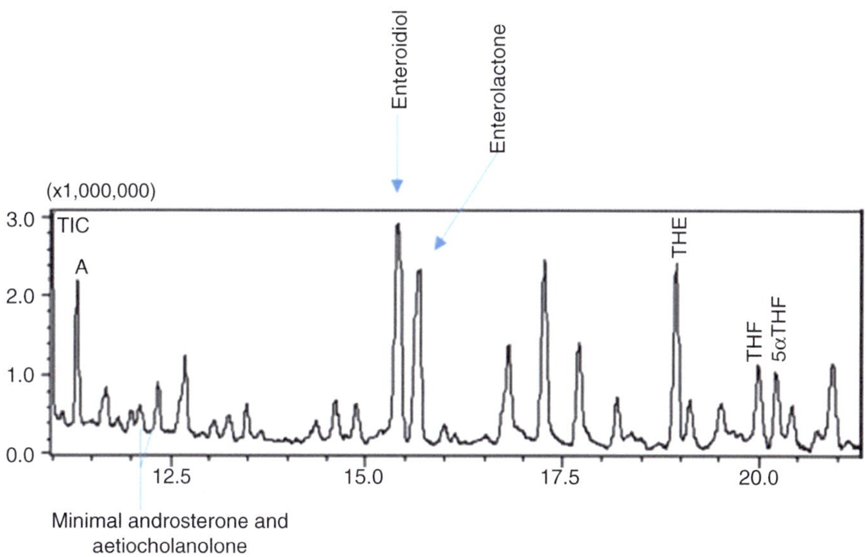

Fig. 3.3 Urine steroid profile from a child preadrenarche shows minimal adrenal androgen metabolites (androsterone and aetiocholanolone) at this stage of development. This spectrum also shows two commonly found dietary components, enterodiol and enterolactone, derived from lignans. 'A' denotes the internal standard, androstanediol

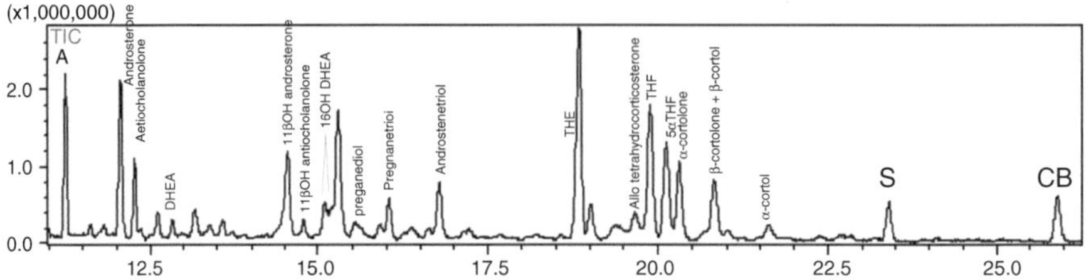

Fig. 3.4 Urine steroid profile from an adult male. Adrenal androgens, androsterone, aetiocholanolone, DHEA and 16α-OH DHEA are much more evident in this profile. A, S and CB denote the internal standards androstanediol, stigmasterol and cholesterol butyrate, respectively

Table 3.2 Steroids that are found in a normal urine steroid profile outside the neonatal period, retention times (methylene units, MU) of their MO-TMS derivatives and relevant ions (see appendix for spectra)

Steroid	Trivial name	MU	Ions
5α-Androstan-3α-ol-17-one	Androsterone	25.11	270, 360
5β-Androstan-3α-ol-17-one	Aetiocholanolone	25.28	270, 360
5-Androsten-3β-ol-17-one	DHEA	25.75	268, 358
5α-Androstan-3α,11β-diol-17-one	11β-OH androsterone	25.95	448, 358
5β-Androstan-3α,11β-diol-17-one	11β-OH aetiocholanolone	25.95	448, 358
5-Androsten-3β,16α-ol-17-one	16α-OHDHEA	27.38, 27.42	266, 446
5β-Pregnan-3α,20α-diol	Pregnanediol	27.64	117, 269
5β-Pregnan-3α,17,20α-triol	Pregnanetriol	28.00	255, 435
5-Androsten-3β,16α,17β-triol	Androstenetriol	28.46	432, 239
5β-Pregan-3α,17,21-triol-11,20-dione	THE	29.65	578, 488
5α-Pregnan-3α,21-diol-11, 20-dione	Allo-tetrahydrocorticosterone	30.00, 30.16	188, 474
5β-Pregnan-3α,11,17,21-tetrol-20-one	THF	30.24	652, 562
5α-Pregnan-3α,11,17,21-tetrol-20-one	5α THF	30.39	652, 562
5β-Pregnan-3α,17,20α,21-tetrol-11-one	α-Cortolone	30.51	449, 359
5β-Pregnan-3α,17,20β,21-tetrol-11-one and 5β-Pregnan-3α,11β,17,20,21-pentol	β-Cortolone + β-cortol	30.73	449, 359
5β-Pregnan-3α,11β,17,20α,21-pentol	α-Cortol	31.20	523, 343

3.7.1 Pregnancy and the Menstrual Cycle

Oestrogens are not usually visible in the steroid profile except in pregnancy where concentrations of oestriol rise throughout gestation. Pregnanediol, derived from progesterone, is also elevated (Fig. 3.5). Females may also exhibit marked changes to pregnanediol and pregnanetriol through the menstrual cycle with the highest levels seen in the luteal phase.

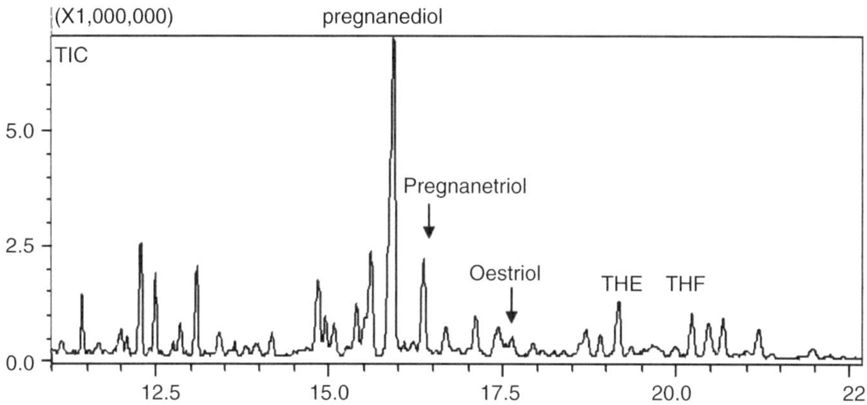

Fig. 3.5 Changes in urine steroid profile in pregnancy. Pregnanediol (from progesterone) reaches extremely high concentrations. Oestriol can be identified by selective ion monitoring using ions at 504 and 386

Table 3.3 Reference range for neonatal steroids (up to 1 month of age)

Neonatal (<1 month old)	ug/24 h
16-α-hydroxy DHEA	200 (40–870)
16-β-hydroxy DHEA	120 (20–380)
16-Oxoandrostenediol + 15,16-dihydroxy DHEA	220 (70–1140)
Androstenetriol	160 (30–500)
16-α,18-dihydroxy DHEA	360 (70–1270)
16-α-hydroxypregnenolone	350 (80–1400)
21-Hydroxypregnenolone	(10–100)
Pregnanetriol	(<50)
Tetrahydrocortisone (THE)	90 (20–290)
α cortolone	10 (<180)
6-α-hydroxy THE	60 (10–300)
β cortolone	20 (<70)
6-Hydroxy-20-α-cortolone	10 (<30)
6-Hydroxy-20-β-cortolone	30 (<140)
1-Hydroxy-20-β-cortolone	20 (<80)

Results are in µg/24 h and represent median and range

3.7.2 Liver Disease

The ratio of 20-hydroxy/20-oxo cortisol metabolites is elevated in chronic liver disease that may be due to increased liver activity of 20-reductases or decreased A ring reduction.

3.7.3 Reference Ranges

Tables 3.3, 3.4 and 3.5 give reference ranges for urine steroid metabolites found in neonates (less than 1 month of age), children and adults.

Table 3.4 Normal values of adrenal steroid metabolites in females

Females	2 years	4 years	6 years	8 years	9 years	10 years	12 years	Adult females
Androsterone	<10	<50	30–100	10–150	30–300	100–400	200–700	260–1270
Aetiocholanolone	<10	<50	30–100	10–120	30–300	150–400	200–500	270–1390
Dehydroepiandrosterone (DHEA)	<10	<20	<50	<100	<100	<200	10–400	<50–970
11-hydroxyandrosterone	<50	10–120	50–150	50–200	50–400	50–400	100–600	130–680
11-hydroxyaetiocholanolone	<20	10–80	50–200	50–200	50–200	50–250	50–300	<50–200
16α-hydroxy-DHEA	<80	<20	10–200	10–200	10–200	10–200	20–500	<50–510
Pregnanediol	<10	<20	<30	<30	<30	<30	20–600	<50–2110
Pregnanetriol	<50	<50	<50	<50	<50	<50	20–100	<50–480
Androstenetriol	<80	<70	<50	<50	<50	<50	20–200	<50–510
THE	50–250	200–800	300–1000	400–1200	300–1500	500–1300	500–1500	980–3240
THF	10–150	50–250	50–300	100–400	100–500	200–550	200–800	440–1610
α-THF	20–300	100–700	100–700	100–800	100–600	200–900	200–1100	160–640
α-cortolone	<50	50–250	50–250	50–300	50–400	50–700	200–900	310–1330
β-cortol + β-cortolone	<50	50–250	50–250	50–250	50–600	50–500	100–500	350–1110
α-cortol	<20	<50	<50	<50	10–160	50–250	20–200	130–350
Total cortisol metabolites	300–900	630–1730	820–2160	1000–2730	900–3000	1600–3600	2650–4640	2630–7300
Total androgen metabolites	<80	<80	40–170	90–140	90–450	260–780	500–1400	570–3280

Values given are in μg/24 h (minimum and maximum)

Table 3.5 Normal values of adrenal steroid metabolites in males

Males	2 years	4 years	6 years	8 years	9 years	10 years	12 years	Adult males
Androsterone	<10	<50	20–150	10–100	30–400	100–600	100–1250	1040–1620
Aetiocholanolone	<10	<50	10–200	10–120	30–300	150–550	100–1000	620–2030
Dehydroepiandrosterone (DHEA)	<10	<20	<100	<100	<100	<200	10–500	<50–1110
11-hydroxyandrosterone	<50	10–120	50–200	50–200	50–350	50–400	200–700	450–780
11-hydroxyaetiocholanolone	<20	13–80	50–200	50–200	50–200	50–250	50–400	<50–310
16α-hydroxy-DHEA	<80	<20	10–200	<30	<30	10–200	20–500	130–400
Pregnanediol	<10	<20	<30	<50	<50	<50	20–100	80–220
Pregnanetriol	<50	<50	<50	<50	<50	<50	20–100	110–520
Androstenetriol	<80	<70	<50	<50	<50	<50	20–250	290–600
THE	50–250	200–800	300–1000	400–1200	450–1250	500–1300	500–2000	1600–3330
THF	10–150	50–250	50–300	100–400	80–450	200–500	200–900	600–1420
αTHF	20–300	100–700	100–800	100–900	150–500	200–900	200–1100	380–910
α-cortolone	<50	50–250	50–250	50–300	50–600	50–700	200–800	220–1100
β-cortolone + β-cortol	<50	50–250	25–250	50–250	50–450	50–500	100–600	410–1370
α-cortol	<20	<50	13–50	13–50	10–100	50–200	20–200	100–450
Total cortisol metabolites	300–900	630–1730	820–2160	1000–2730	1200–3200	1600–3600	2650–4640	4070–7490
Total androgen metabolites	<80	<80	40–300	30–470	130–1000	220–1200	280–1290	2150–3590

Values given are in μg/24 h (minimum and maximum)

Further Reading

Derivation of Mass Spectra

Shackleton CHL. Mass spectrometry: application to steroid and peptide research. Endocr Rev. 1985;6:441–86.

Historical Context

Shackleton CHL. Profiling steroid hormones and urinary steroids. J Chrom B: Biomedical Sciences and Applications. 1986;379:91–156.

Complimentary Role of LC/MS–MS

Krone N, Hughes BA, Lavery GG, Stewart PM, Arlt W, Shackleton CHL. Gas chromatography/mass spectrometry (GC/MS) remains a pre-eminent discovery tool in clinical steroid investigations even in the era of fast liquid chromatography tandem mass spectrometry (LC/MS/MS). J Steroid Biochem Mol Biol. 2010;121(3-5):496–504.

21-Hydroxylase Deficiency

4

Gill Rumsby

4.1 Introduction

The steroid 21-hydroxylase (CYP21) enzyme catalyses the introduction of a hydroxyl group at the carbon 21 position of progesterone and 17-hydroxyprogesterone (17OHP) to produce 11-deoxycorticosterone and 11-deoxycortisol, respectively (Fig. 4.1). Thus, the enzyme plays an essential role in the synthesis of both mineralocorticoids and glucocorticoids.

This microsomal enzyme is a member of the cytochrome P450 family of mixed-function oxidases. NADPH provides reducing equivalents for the reaction, and these are transferred to CYP21 via the FMN moiety of cytochrome P450 oxidoreductase (POR), a cofactor for at least 50 other enzymes including the steroid 17α-hydroxylase (CYP17) enzyme. CYP21 has similar affinity for its primary substrates progesterone and 17OHP, but, unlike CYP17, cytochrome b5 does not appear to have a stimulatory effect on the enzyme. CYP21 has been shown to be expressed in all three zones of the adrenal in the adult, but the enzyme is mainly active in the zona glomerulosa and fasciculata, while in the fetus, it is predominantly in the transitional and fetal zones with only a small but detectable amount in the definitive zone. Enzyme synthesis is under the regulation of adrenocorticotropic hormone (ACTH) mediated by the action of adenylyl cyclase. Transcriptional regulators include steroidogenic factor 1 (SF1) and the cyclic AMP response element-binding protein, CREB.

Deficiency of CYP21 is the most common cause of congenital adrenal hyperplasia (CAH) with an incidence in the region of 1:15,000 and carrier frequency of 1/60. This form of CAH is characterised by failure of cortisol and aldosterone synthesis in conjunction with excess adrenal androgen production that is metabolised to testosterone in peripheral tissues. Exposure of the affected female to excess androgen

G. Rumsby
Department of Clinical Biochemistry, University College London Hospitals, London, UK
e-mail: gill.rumsby@nhs.net

G. Rumsby, G. M. Woodward (eds.), *Disorders of Steroidogenesis*,
https://doi.org/10.1007/978-3-319-96364-8_4

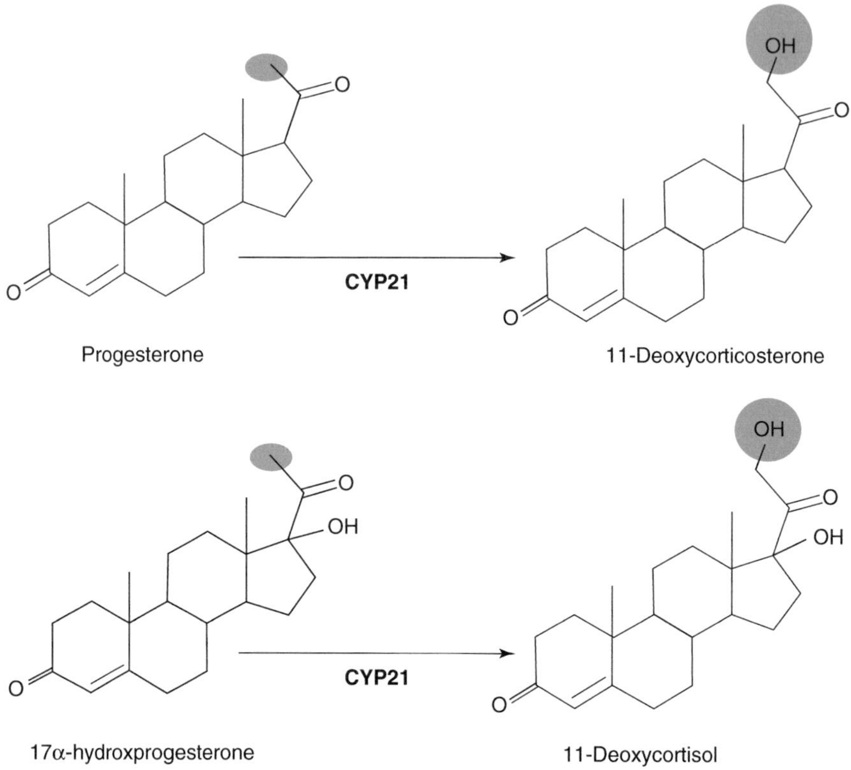

Fig. 4.1 CY21 catalyses the hydroxylation of progesterone and 17-hydroxyprogesterone to 11-deoxycorticosterone and 11-deoxycortisol, respectively

in utero leads to ambiguous external genitalia ranging in severity from clitoromegaly to labial fusion. In some cases, the degree of virilisation is so severe that incorrect gender assignment is made. Males have normal genital development, and the disorder may therefore not be recognised at birth unless presenting in a renal salt-losing crisis.

Failure to synthesise cortisol lifts the negative feedback system on the hypothalamus and pituitary with unregulated ACTH secretion leading to an increase in cell number and size of the adrenal gland. Chronic ACTH stimulation also leads to an increase in transcription of all the enzymes in the cortisol pathway. Decreased aldosterone synthesis underlies renal salt-losing with renin rising in response to fluid loss.

The source of androgens in CYP21 deficiency is in part the result of increased flow down the Δ5 pathway from 17-hydroxypregnenolone to dehydroepiandrosterone (DHEA). This step, catalysed by CYP17, is normally low throughout early childhood but increases in response to increased expression of cytochrome b5 in the zona reticularis that underpins the onset of adrenarche. The Δ4 pathway is only likely to play a minor role as, even at high 17OHP concentrations, the reaction is unfavourable. A third pathway, the so-called 'backdoor' pathway (Fig. 4.2), has also

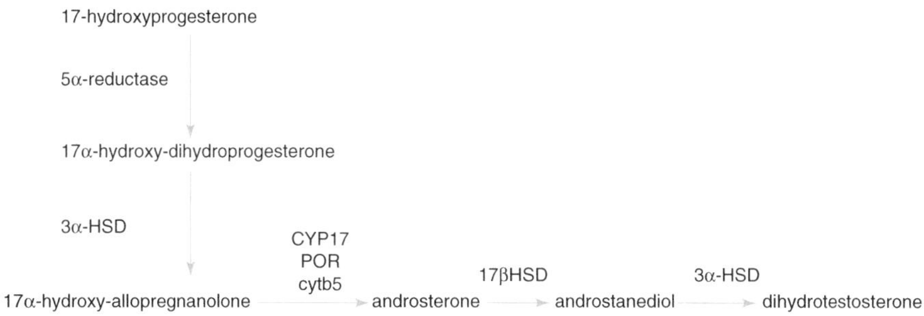

Fig. 4.2 Backdoor pathway of androgen production from 17OHP. 3αHSD 3α-hydroxysteroid dehydrogenase, CYP17 17α-hydroxylase, POR P450 oxidoreductase, cytb5 cytochrome b5, 17βHSD 17β-hydroxysteroid dehydrogenase

been described that produces dihydrotestosterone, a potent androgen, via 17α-hydroxyallopregnanolone (5α-pregnane-3α,17α-diol-20-one). While 17OHP is a poor substrate for CYP17, it is a better substrate for 5α-reductase, and the excess 17OHP can therefore be reduced to 17α-hydroxydihydroprogesterone, followed by reduction of the ketone group at C3 to 17α-hydroxyallopregnanolone in a step catalysed by 3α-hydroxysteroid dehydrogenase types 1 and 3 (AKR1C4 and AKR1C2, respectively). The next step, cleavage of the side chain, is facilitated by CYP17 with the formation of androsterone that is subsequently reduced at carbon 17 by 17β-hydroxysteroid dehydrogenase (one of the AKR1C enzymes) to androstanediol. The final oxidation step to dihydrotestosterone is potentially catalysed by one of the 3α-hydroxysteroid dehydrogenase enzymes.

Support for the backdoor pathway is the finding of a mismatch between high serum 17OHP and relatively low androstenedione and testosterone in virilised CAH patients with raised urinary androsterone relative to aetiocholanolone, the latter a product of the classical pathway only. In addition, 17α-hydroxyallopregnanolone is a significant urinary metabolite in CYP21 CAH. Mutations affecting AKR1C2, one of the 3αHSD enzymes, have been shown to cause a 46XY disorder of sex development suggesting that this pathway may be of particular importance for normal human male sexual differentiation.

Another adrenal androgen, 11β-hydroxyandrostenedione, and its 11-oxo metabolite, have also been implicated as androgen precursors, in particular of 11-oxotestosterone, a steroid with similar affinity for the androgen receptor as testosterone. The 11-oxo-C19 steroids are purely adrenal in origin and are products of androstenedione metabolism, but in CYP21 deficiency, 11β-hydroxyandrostenedione can also arise from the metabolism of 21-deoxycortisol, produced by the action of 11-hydroxylase on 17OHP (Fig. 4.3). The urinary metabolite of 11β-hydroxyandrostenedione, 11β-hydroxyandrosterone, represents the dominant serum (adrenal) androgen in children with CAH.

Extra-adrenal sources of 21-hydroxylation are recognised leading to some 21-hydroxylated metabolites even in complete CYP21 deficiency. Both CYP3A4 and CYP2C19 can utilise progesterone but not 17OHP, while CYP2D6 can

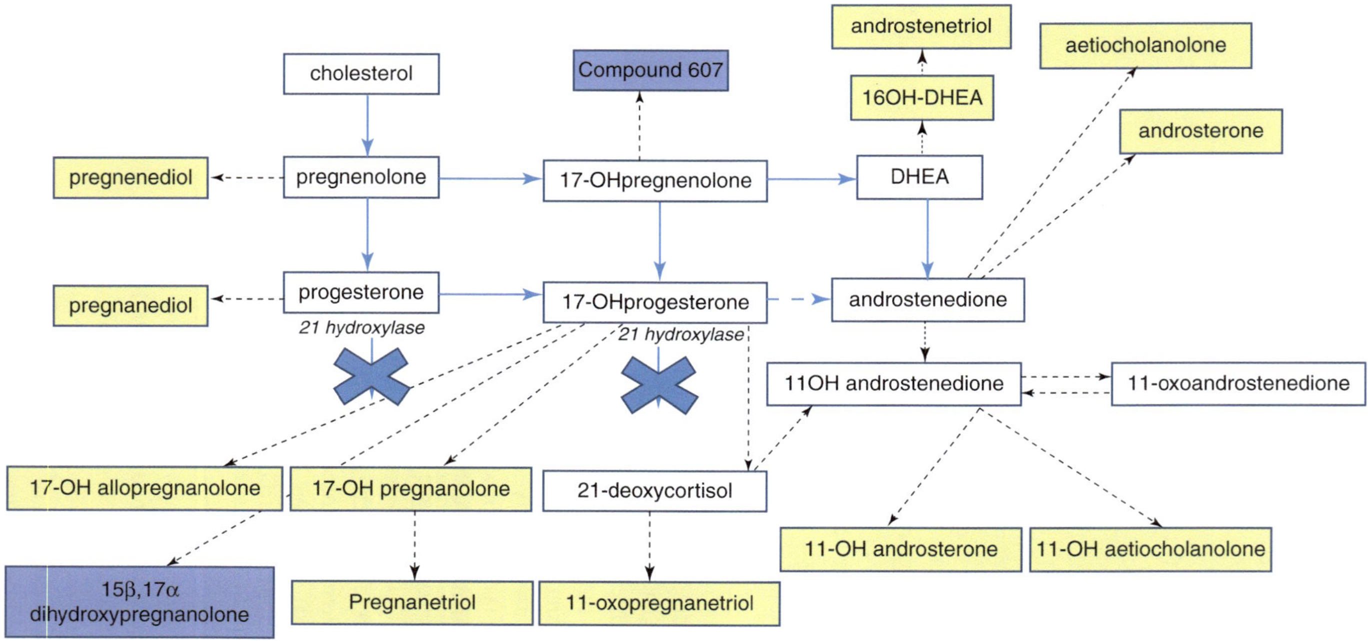

Fig. 4.3 Origin of urinary metabolites seen in CYP21 deficiency. Neonatal metabolites are shown in blue, the others in yellow

21-hydroxylate 17OHP. These enzymes may contribute to a decrease in the requirements for mineralocorticoid replacement in some adults.

4.2 Presentation

The disorder is historically described as either 'classical' or 'nonclassical' essentially reflecting the age of onset and, within these categories, as salt-losing and simple virilising. These classifications have little merit as all arise from mutations within the *CYP21A2* gene and the disease is a continuum but in essence reflect the impact of these mutations on enzyme activity. Newborn babies may present in a salt-losing crisis but not usually before 5 days by which time they have most likely been discharged from hospital. Ambiguity of the external genitalia may be evident, particularly in females, prompting earlier investigation. Males without salt-losing crises typically present later in childhood with symptoms reflecting excess androgen output, e.g. pubic hair growth, aggressive behaviour, and are subsequently found to have advanced bone age. Milder forms of disease, the result of less severe mutations, often present later in life in females with hirsutism, oligomenorrhoea, recurrent miscarriage or severe acne. In some males, the diagnosis may only be made after family studies are performed (cryptic disease) or following investigation for bilateral testicular growths that turn out to be testicular adrenal rests (TARTS). The origin of TARTs is not entirely clear. They either originate from adrenocortical cells from the common gonadal-adrenal primordium or from totipotent embryonic cells expressing markers of the adrenal cortex and Leydig cells. In either case, their growth is promoted by chronic ACTH stimulation and to a certain extent reflects poor disease control in males.

4.3 Genetics

CYP21A2 is found on the short arm of chromosome 6 within the HLA class III region. The gene is located some 30 kilobases (kb) downstream of a pseudogene, *CYP21A1P*, that shares over 98% nucleotide sequence homology but contains a number of changes that render the transcript defective. The pseudogene and *CYP21A2* are found at the 3′ ends of the genes for the fourth component of complement, *C4A* and *C4B*, respectively, and it appears that this whole region arose as a result of ancestral duplication. On the opposite strand of DNA is a gene for tenascin X, encoding an extracellular matrix protein, deficiency of which can lead to a form of Ehlers–Danlos syndrome. Thus, contiguous gene deletions affecting this locus can lead to a spectrum of disorders.

About one-quarter of mutations arise from partial deletions of *CYP21A2* arising from misalignment of the genes in meiosis and the formation of a chimaera containing the 5′ end of the pseudogene and the 3′ end of *CYP21A2*. This hybrid gene lacks the correct promoter and also has some deleterious sequence in the 5′ end and is therefore non-functional. The overall effect of this recombination event is a loss of

30 kb containing *C4B* and the 5′ end of *CYP21A2*. The reciprocal product of this crossover event is an allele with three genes, one of which is a hybrid, this time with the 5′ end of *CYP21A2* and the 3′ end of the pseudogene. It is non-functional but can lead to potential problems with DNA diagnostic methodologies.

A significant number of other mutations also appear to derive from the pseudogene and may have arisen by a process of gene conversion where *CYP21A2* takes on some of the sequence of the pseudogene, but the number of genes remains the same. As multiple gene conversion events can occur on the same allele, it can lead to diagnostic uncertainty. Family studies are therefore essential to confirm that the mutations are present on different alleles.

In addition to the common 30 kb deletion, three other mutations are worthy of note. One of these, a C>G change in intron 2 (c.293-13C>G), occurs in approximately 20–25% cases and leads to missplicing of intron 2 incorporating an extra 13 bp into the transcript and a resulting frame shift. This mutation is typically associated with the early-onset, salt-wasting form of disease reflecting its severity. The p.Ile172Asn missense change that occurs in 17%, particularly simple virilising forms, has approximately 3–7% activity in vitro. In contrast, the p.Val281Leu change is found at high frequency (55%) in late-presenting forms of the disease. This mutant protein demonstrates significant activity in vitro, up to 20% with progesterone and 50% with 17-hydroxyprogesterone although more recent studies indicate that these are perhaps an overestimate. Considerable effort has been made to assign a genotype–phenotype relationship in this disorder, but it is not altogether successful. The more severe changes, that is, null mutations, do tend to present early and have renal salt-losing, but there are exceptions in all cases.

Genetic testing has made possible a reliable prenatal diagnosis for this disorder using either mutation analysis or linkage analysis to HLA markers.

4.4 Diagnosis

In any child suspected of having CAH or adrenal failure from any cause, it is preferable to take blood for cortisol and 17-hydroxyprogesterone in addition to a urine sample for steroid profile prior to treatment with steroids. In the case of ambiguous genitalia, a blood sample is also needed for karyotype analysis to determine the genetic sex and establish whether the child is a virilised female or under-virilised male. As rapid fluid replacement is required in these situations, it may be necessary to do investigations after treatment has been implemented in which case the clinician should be alerted to the fact that abnormal metabolites may be suppressed to the normal range. In this case, the response of cortisol and 17-hydroxyprogesterone to ACTH stimulation can be assessed. Recent changes in cortisol methodologies mean that the cut-offs for adequate adrenal function are very method dependent and may well be lower than previously seen with immunoassay methods. However, 17OHP, if measured by a specific method, for example, gas chromatography–mass spectrometry or liquid chromatography–mass spectrometry, that has minimal interference from fetal adrenal steroids, should be >60 nmol/L in an affected child and is typically >200 nmol/L. Obligate carriers of the disease may achieve values of up to 30 nmol/L following ACTH stimulation, and in some cases, slight elevations in 17OHP can occur in 11-hydroxylase and 3β-hydroxysteroid dehydrogenase deficiencies but not usually to levels that cause diagnostic confusion.

A urine steroid profile taken in the first 3 days of life can be difficult to interpret as maternal and placental-derived steroids may still be present, but after that time, in the untreated patient, there is a characteristic increase of 17OHP metabolites: 17-hydroxypregnanolone, pregnanetriol and 11-oxopregnanetriol. In the neonate, there is also 15,17-dihydroxypregnanolone and 3β,16α,17α-trihydroxy-5α-pregnane-7,20-dione ('compound 607'), the latter seen in the sulphate conjugate fraction. These markers may be suppressed if treatment has been given. If assessing after ACTH stimulation, the urine needs to be collected some 4–5 h after ACTH to allow time for the metabolites to form and to be excreted into urine.

In patients with some residual enzyme activity, cortisol synthesis may be maintained but at the expense of excessive adrenal androgen production leading to symptoms of virilisation as previously described. Cortisol response to ACTH stimulation may be substantial in late-presenting cases, albeit at the low end of normal. There will, however, be an abnormal response by 17OHP to greater than 60 nmol/L, even though this analyte may be initially unremarkable and possibly even within the reference range. As these patients are typically untreated while under investigation, a urine steroid profile is helpful to confirm the presence of the characteristic abnormal metabolites in an unstimulated sample along with those of cortisol. Carriers of CYP21 deficiency do not show any abnormality in urine steroids.

4.5 Case Study

The second child of unrelated parents was born at home. On day 12 the child refused feeds, was vomiting and became floppy. On presentation in the emergency department, serum sodium was 120 mmol/L and potassium 6.0 mmol/L. Fluid replacement was commenced. On examination clitoromegaly was noted raising the suspicion of CAH. Blood was taken for serum cortisol, and a urine collection begun. Steroid replacement was commenced. On review, an additional sample was taken for 17OHP.

The karyotype was 46XX consistent with a virilised female infant. Serum cortisol on the initial sample was 100 nmol/L suggestive of adrenal failure, but the 17OHP was only 8.5 nmol/L making CYP21 deficiency unlikely but did not exclude other forms of CAH. The urine steroid profile showed the characteristic elevation of 17OHP metabolites and the neonatal metabolite compound 607 consistent with CYP21 deficiency. A subsequent Synacthen stimulation test showed an abnormal response of both 17OHP and cortisol (Table 4.1), and it was concluded that the initial 17OHP had been taken after treatment leading to a false-negative result. The timing of samples relative to treatment is often not communicated to the laboratory, and a comment about the possibility of false-negative results on treatment should be included on the report (Fig. 4.4).

Table 4.1 Response of cortisol and 17OHP to ACTH stimulation in a child with CYP21 deficiency

Time (min)	Cortisol (nmol/L)	17OHP (nmol/L)
0	140	51
60	150	360
	Normal response: >415 nmol/L	Normal response: <10 nmol/L CYP21 heterozygotes:<30 nmol/L

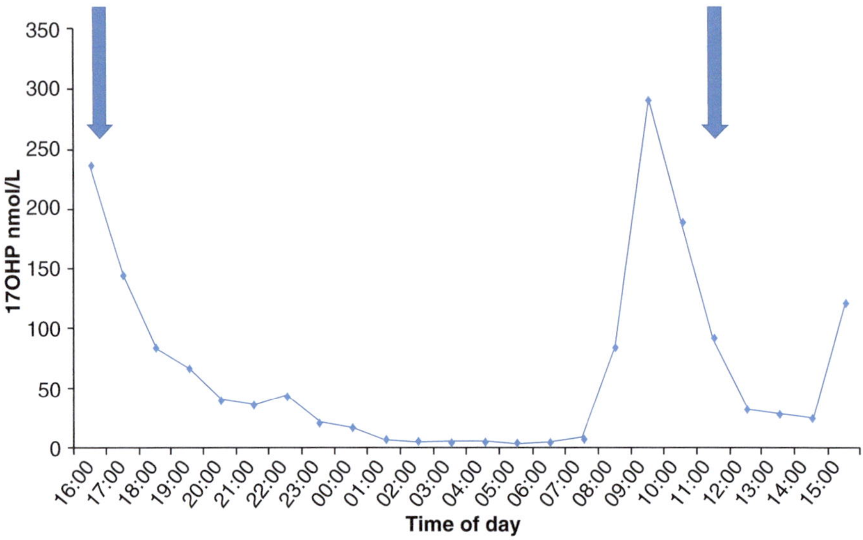

Fig. 4.4 Effect of treatment (arrows) on 17OHP results showing the possibility of false-negative result if the sample is taken after treatment is implemented

The need for lifelong treatment of this disease justifies the use of two different biochemical tests for its diagnosis.

Genetic testing was subsequently carried out, and the child was found to be homozygous for the intron 2 splice site mutation.

4.6 Steroid Profile

A huge number of steroid metabolites arising from 17OHP and progesterone have been identified in CYP21 deficiency in the neonate (see Further Reading section). These compounds make the profile considerably more complex than that for any other form of CAH and highlight the presence of numerous pathways of steroid metabolism that are active in early life. The CYP21-deficient neonatal profile is characterised by an excess of 16-hydroxypregnenolone to 16α-hydroxyDHEA (16α-OH DHEA) in the sulphate fraction (Fig. 4.5) with values 3–5 times those seen in the normal infant. This finding is possibly related to the faster involution of

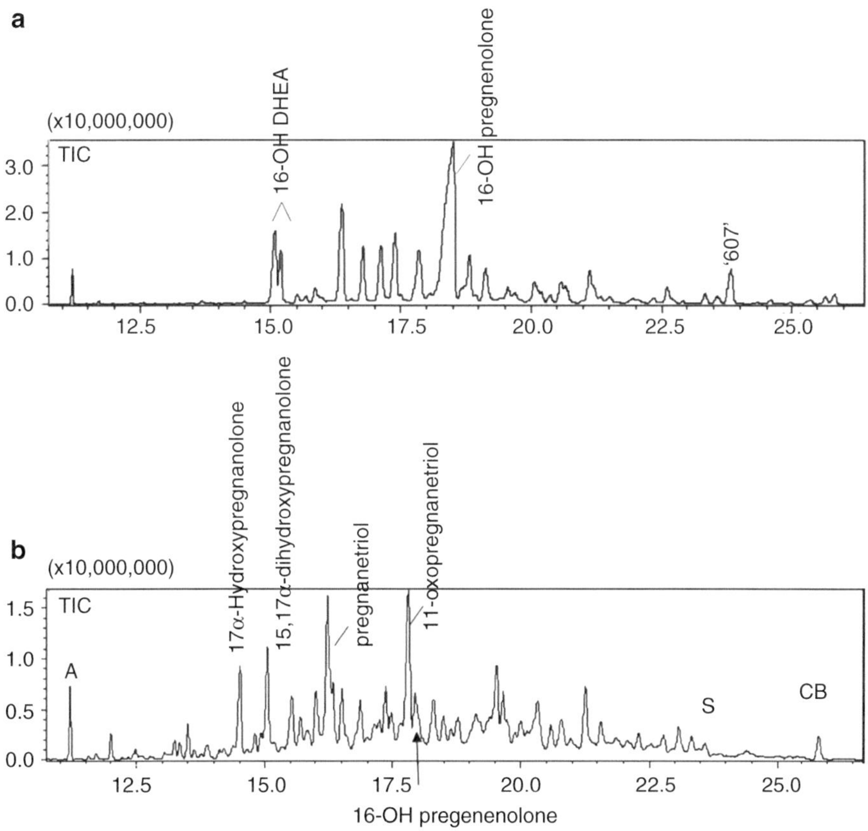

Fig. 4.5 Urine steroid profile from a neonate with CYP21 deficiency. (**a**) Illustrates the 30+ (sulphate) fraction and (**b**) the 0–30 fractions (free steroid and glucuronide). Note the elevated 16-hydroxypregnenolone relative to 16α-OH DHEA and the '607' peaks in the sulphate fraction that are characteristic of CYP21 deficiency. The other peaks in the neonatal profile are as described in Chap. 3. The glucuronide fraction (**b**) in this case shows the neonatal-specific, 15,17-dihydroxypregnanolone metabolite, along with the three metabolites associated with CYP21 deficiency at all ages: 17-hydroxypregnanolone, pregnanetriol and 11-oxopregnanetriol; the latter is often not quite so marked in the neonatal form of disease. No cortisol metabolites are present. A, S and CB in (**b**) denote the internal standards

the fetal adrenal in patients induced by activation of the renin–angiotensin system by renal salt-wasting. It is, however, less extreme than that seen in 17α-hydroxylase deficiency where DHEA metabolites are even lower, if produced at all.

Two important neonatal metabolites are compound 607 and 15,17-dihydroxypregnanolone (Fig. 4.5 and Table 4.3). Compound 607 is thought to arise from hepatic metabolism of 17-hydroxypregnenolone by hydroxylation reactions at C16 and C7, the latter catalysed by CYP7A1. The C7-hydroxyl is then oxidised by the action of 11β-hydroxysteroid dehydrogenase 1 followed by 5α-reduction. The metabolite is found in the sulphate fraction and has been shown to be present in the first 3–4 weeks of life, with maximum amounts around day 4 of life. There is considerable variability in output of this compound that correlates with serum 17OHP. There is some anecdotal evidence that it is not wholly specific for CYP21, but it does not appear to be present in any other neonatal form of CAH to date and has proven extremely useful for the diagnosis of neonatal CYP21 deficiency in conjunction with other markers, occurring in part of the profile less cluttered with other metabolites.

Hydroxylation at C15 is a normal pathway in the neonate, and therefore the finding of 15,17-dihydroxypregnanolone simply reflects a neonatal metabolic pathway for the metabolism of excess 17OHP. The ratio of this metabolite over total cortisol metabolites (i.e. 15,17 DHP ×100/(cortisol, cortisone, α-cortolone and β-cortolone)) has been used as a diagnostic ratio for CYP21 in the neonate with values from 47 to 1627 found in the first month of life compared to less than 17 in unaffected neonates. 11-Oxopregnanetriol, a metabolite of 21-deoxycortisol, has also shown good discrimination for the diagnosis of CYP21 deficiency when expressed as a ratio to the neonatal cortisol metabolite, 6-hydroxytetrahydrocortisone; ratios were some eight times higher than seen in normal neonates and preterm infants. Determination of these ratios in the first few days of life may, however, be compromised because some of the cortisol metabolites will derive from the maternal circulation.

There are multiple hydroxylated metabolites of pregnanes and pregnene metabolites ranging from di- to hexa-hydroxylated. These can be recognised by selected ion plots of the M-31 ions (Table 4.2). Untreated neonates with CYP21 deficiency have been shown to produce significant amounts of the pregnanepentol-20-ones, 1β,3α,6α,17α,21-pentahydroxy-5β-pregnane-2-one and 1β,3α,6α,16α17α-pentahydroxy-5β-pregnane-2-one characterised by ions at 740 (M-31) with a base peak at 147. If treatment has been given, an additional peak of 3α,6α,11β, 17α,21-pentahydroxy-5β-pregnane-20-one (6α-hydroxytetrahydrocortisol) appears between them.

Treatment prior to taking the urine sample may be obvious from a very large peak of free cortisol (Fig. 4.6) present in the chromatogram or the presence of characteristic markers of prednisolone (Fig. 4.7). Such treatment will make interpretation difficult if not impossible as abnormal markers will be suppressed and a fresh sample should be requested off treatment.

The usual markers of CYP21 deficiency in older patients, 11-oxopregnanetriol and pregnanetriol, are present in the neonate but account for less than 10% of the

Table 4.2 GC–MS ion plots for -OTMS derivatives of multiple hydroxylation products of 20-oxo pregnanes and pregnenes seen in CYP21 deficiency

	Pregnane	Pregnene
-Diolone	476	474
-Triolone	564	562
-Tetrolone	652	650
-Pentolone	740	738
-Hexolone	828	826

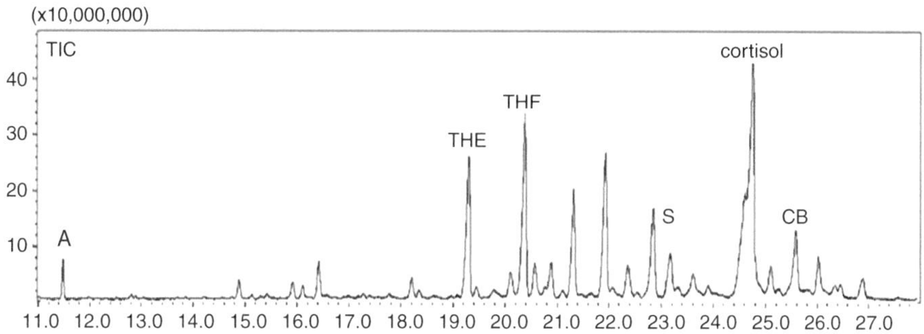

Fig. 4.6 Effect of hydrocortisone on urine steroid profile. Free cortisol in this particular case is obvious, and cortisol metabolites are correspondingly high. A, S and CB are the internal standards

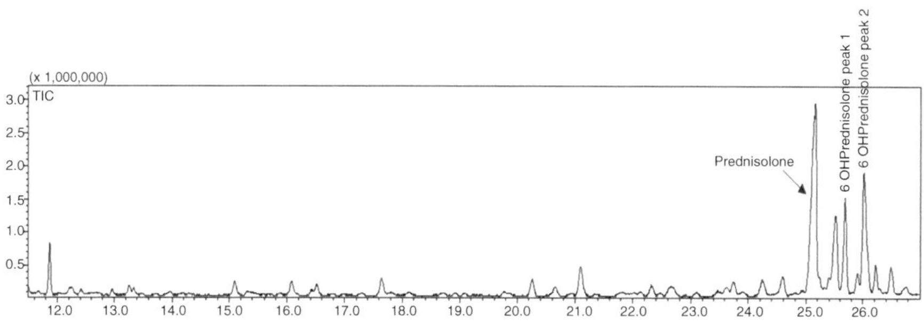

Fig. 4.7 Effect of prednisolone on urine steroid profile. Such treatment can lead to suppression of other adrenal steroids

total 17OHP metabolites because of metabolism of 17OHP by other routes (Table 4.3).

Outside the neonatal period, the three major metabolites pregnanetriol, 17-hydroxypregnanolone and 11-oxopregnanetriol are clearly evident (Fig. 4.8). The latter is formed by the action of 11β-hydroxylase on 17-hydroxyprogesterone followed by oxidation of the hydroxyl group at C11 by 11β-hydroxysteroid dehydrogenase and reduction of the C-20 ketone group to hydroxyl by 20α-hydroxysteroid dehydrogenase (Fig. 4.3). Cortisol metabolites will be reduced although in the case of late-presenting forms of CYP21 deficiency may still be present in significant amounts.

4.7 Treatment

The treatment for CYP21 deficiency is glucocorticoid and mineralocorticoid replacement along with salt supplements as seen for adrenal insufficiency but with the added additional problem of the need to minimise excessive androgen

Table 4.3 Relevant steroids found in CYP21 deficiency, retention times (methylene units, MU) of their MO-TMS derivatives and characteristic ions (see appendix for spectra)

Steroid	Trivial name	MU	Characteristic ions
3α,17α-Dihydroxy-5β-pregnan-20-one	17-OHpregnanolone	27.00	476, 188
5α-Androstan-3α,11β-diol-17-one	11β-Hydroxyandrosterone	27.00	448, 358
5β-Androstan-3α,11β-diol-17-one	11β-Hydroxyaetiocholanolone	27.18	448, 358
3α,17α-Dihydroxy-5α-pregnan-20-one	Allo 17-OHpregnanolone	27.54	476, 188
5β-Pregnane-3α,17α,20α-triol	Pregnanetriol	28.21	435, 255
3α,17α,20α-Trihydroxy-5β-pregnan-11-one	11-Oxopregnanetriol	29.34	449, 359
Neonatal metabolites			
3α,15β,17α-Trihydroxy-5β-pregnan-20-one	15,17-Dihydroxypregnanolone	27.39	564, 258
5-Androsten-3β,16α-diol-17-one	16αOH DHEA*	27.63/27.72	266, 446
3α,15β,17α-Trihydroxy-5β-pregnan-20-one	15,17-Dihydroxypregnanolone	27.39	564, 258
5-Pregnen-3β,16α-diol-20-one	16-OHpregnenolone*	29.38	474, 384
5-Pregnen-3β,15β,17α,20α-tetrol		29.97	521
5β-Pregnan-3α,6,17,21-tetrol-11,20-dione	6OH-THE	30.80	666, 576
3β,16α,17α-Trihydroxy-5α-pregnane-7,20-dione	607*	32.58	607

Metabolites with asterisk (*) denote those found primarily in the sulphate fraction

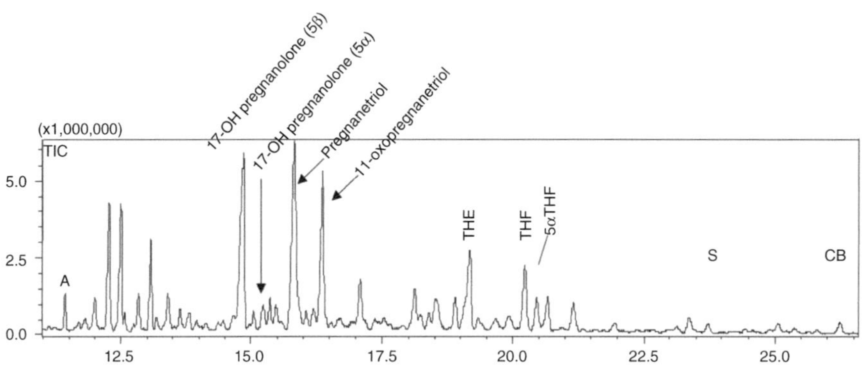

Fig. 4.8 CYP21 deficiency outside the neonatal period showing the three urinary metabolites of 17OHP: 17α-hydroxypregnanolone (5β and 5α metabolites), pregnanetriol and 11-oxopregnanetriol. Some cortisol metabolites are also present. A, S and CB denote the internal standards

production in females and prepubertal males with the disorder. A satisfactory outcome can be difficult to achieve as undertreatment leads to androgen-induced rapid growth but eventual short stature, while overtreatment leads to a Cushingoid picture.

The usual therapy is with hydrocortisone and fludrocortisone, hydrocortisone in 2–3 divided doses being the glucocorticoid of choice in childhood. Prednisolone and dexamethasone have longer half-lives and are not recommended for the growing child but may be used in adults, particularly those with poor compliance. Treatment is monitored clinically by assessment of growth and by measurement of renin and 17OHP. Subclinical aldosterone insufficiency, as determined by elevated renin, may be present even in those patients who have not had salt-losing episodes and may benefit from mineralocorticoid replacement. As can be seen in Fig. 4.4, 17OHP fluctuates markedly relative to time of treatment, and therefore monitoring needs to be done at a consistent time relative to treatment. The aim is not to suppress 17OHP entirely as this would indicate overtreatment; rather the 17OHP should be slightly outside the reference range. Measurement of the usual serum androgens, androstenedione, DHEAS and testosterone have not been shown to be particularly helpful as markers of androgen excess; DHEAS in particular tends to be lower than controls even in untreated CYP21 deficiency. 11-Hydroxyandrostenedione and its urinary metabolite, 11-β-hydroxyandrosterone, have recently been shown to have some merit for this purpose as it is purely adrenal in origin.

Recently, treatment with the 17α-hydroxylase inhibitor, abiraterone, has been proposed to minimise adrenal androgen synthesis in females with the disease. This drug, primarily used for the inhibition of androgen production in prostatic tissue, may allow a reduction in the hydrocortisone dose.

Patients with persistently high progesterone may experience difficulties with ovulation. In some cases this situation has been overcome by adrenalectomy along with steroid replacement.

Further Reading

Neonatal Metabolism

Christakoudi S, Cowan DA, Taylor DA. Steroids excreted in urine by neonates with 21-hydroxylase deficiency: characterisation, using GC-MS and GC-MS/MS, of the D-ring and side chain structure of pregnanes and pregnenes. Steroids. 2010;75:34–52.

Disease Management

Speiser PW, Azziz R, Baskin LS, et al. Congenital adrenal hyperplasia due to steroid 21-hydroxylase deficiency: an Endocrine Society clinical practice guideline. J Clin Endocrinol Metab. 2010;95(9):4133–60.

Genetics

Wang C, Pallan PS, Zhang W, et al. Functional analysis of human cytochrome P45021A2 variants involved in congenital adrenal hyperplasia. J Biol Chem. 2017;292(26):10767–78.

11β-Hydroxylase Deficiency

5

Gill Rumsby

5.1 Introduction

The 11β-hydroxylase enzyme (CYP11B1) catalyses the final step in cortisol biosynthesis from 11-deoxycortisol to cortisol in the zona fasciculata (Fig. 5.1) under the control of adrenocorticotrophic hormone (ACTH). The enzyme is located on the matrix side of the inner mitochondrial membrane and is a member of the cytochrome P450 group of mixed function oxidases. In common with other mitochondrial P450s, the enzyme utilises molecular oxygen and receives reducing equivalents, that is, electrons, from NADPH via the electron transport protein adrenodoxin reductase, an NADPH-dependent, FAD-containing reductase. These electrons are then donated to adrenodoxin and from there pass to CYP11B1. The enzyme shares significant homology with aldosterone synthase (CYP11B2) with 471 out of 503 amino acids identical. The N-terminal 24-amino-acid signal peptide is cleaved to yield a mature protein of 479 amino acids. In spite of the sequence similarity, CYP11B1 poorly catalyses hydroxylation at the C18 position and completely lacks 18-oxidase activity and thus cannot produce aldosterone. The tertiary structure of the protein has shown that the active site of CYP11B1 is larger than that of CYP11B2 and thus is able to accommodate the larger natural substrate, 11-deoxycortisol, with its additional 17-hydroxyl group. Two arginine residues, Arg448 and Arg384, provide hydrogen bonds to the haem moiety characteristic of P450 cytochrome P450 enzymes and are essential for functional activity.

CYP11B1 deficiency is an autosomal recessive disorder and accounts for 5–8% of cases of congenital adrenal hyperplasia (CAH). The disorder has a prevalence of 1 in 100,000 worldwide although is higher in certain ethnic groups presumably reflecting a smaller gene pool. The disorder can lead to virilisation of the external genitalia of females in utero, the result of diversion of the excess precursors to

G. Rumsby
Department of Clinical Biochemistry, University College London Hospitals, London, UK
e-mail: gill.rumsby@nhs.net

G. Rumsby, G. M. Woodward (eds.), *Disorders of Steroidogenesis*,
https://doi.org/10.1007/978-3-319-96364-8_5

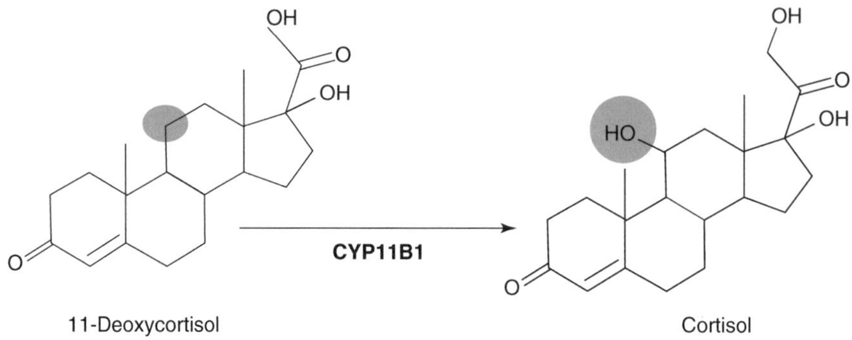

Fig. 5.1 Conversion of 11-deoxycortisol to cortisol catalysed by 11β-hydroxylase (CYP11B1)

adrenal androgen synthesis in a similar manner to that seen in 21-hydroxylase deficiency. Virilisation takes the form of clitoromegaly or clitoral fusion leading to genital ambiguity and in some cases to incorrect gender assignment. As with all forms of virilising CAH, the internal, Müllerian duct-derived organs are unaffected, but the degree of virilisation can lead to significant problems requiring multiple rounds of corrective surgery in later life with variable degrees of success. The excess androgen production is obviously less evident in males at birth, and the disorder may be initially undetected but present later with symptoms of pseudoprecocious puberty (see below). Approximately two-thirds of patients have hypertension thought to be the result of excess precursors with mineralocorticoid activity (Fig. 5.2). Deoxycorticosterone (DOC), the substrate for 11-hydroxylase in the aldosterone pathway, was initially suspected to be the primary culprit, but there is no clear correlation between DOC and hypertension, and it is possible that other metabolites of DOC with mineralocorticoid properties are responsible.

5.2 Presentation

The disease may be suspected in a neonate presenting with genital ambiguity. Although the disorder is classically associated with salt retention, salt-losing may be evident in the neonate and may reflect a variety of causes, so the differential diagnosis must include all forms of CAH in the first instance.

As with other forms of virilising CAH, the excess androgen production may become apparent in young children in terms of rapid growth, premature pubic hair development and aggressive behaviour—symptoms typically described as pseudoprecocious puberty. Blood pressure measurements are notoriously difficult in children and need to be interpreted in relation to age-related controls. Individuals presenting in later life may present with symptoms of androgen excess, for example, hirsutism, irregular periods, or those related to hypertension, for example, headaches, and typically have low renin hypertension. Electrolyte disturbances, for example, decreased serum potassium causing muscle weakness, may also be present.

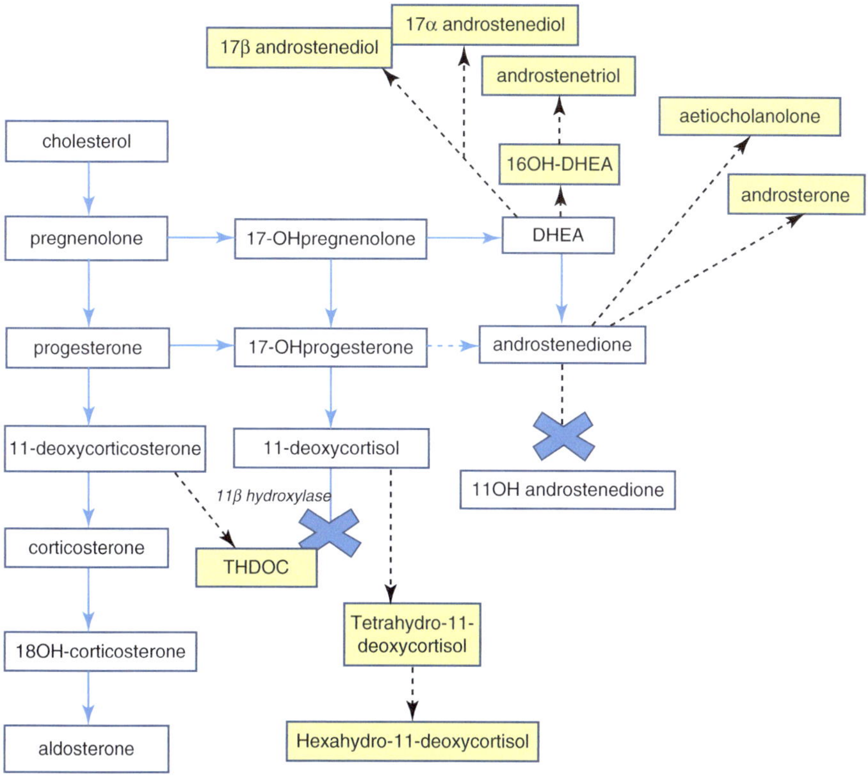

Fig. 5.2 Illustration of the metabolic block caused by CYP11B1 deficiency and origin of the resulting urine steroid metabolites

5.3 Genetics

The recognition that there are two different 11-hydroxylase enzymes, CYP11B1 and CYP11B2, in the zona fasciculata and glomerulosa respectively arose from the description of glucocorticoid remedial hyperaldosteronism (GRA, also known as dexamethasone suppressible aldosteronism), a condition in which aldosterone is synthesised in the zona fasciculata under the regulation of ACTH. This disorder was found to be caused by recombination between the aldosterone synthase gene (*CYP11B2*) and *CYP11B1* leading to a hybrid gene, the 5′ end encoded by *CYP11B1* and the 3′ end by *CYP11B2*. The two genes were subsequently shown to be located in tandem on the long arm of chromosome 8q24.3 approximately 40 kilobases apart and share a high degree of homology with 95% of exonic sequence identical. They differ in two main areas: firstly, the gene promoters—*CYP11B1* is regulated by ACTH and *CYP11B2* by the renin–angiotensin system; secondly, there are coding differences in exons 5 and 6 that account for the inability of *CYP11B1* to encode a protein with 18-hydroxylase and 18-oxidase activities.

The majority of mutations in *CYP11B1* are missense changes or minor deletions. In vitro expression of some of the former has led to a greater understanding of the role of different residues in enzyme function, for example, the previously mentioned p.Arg448His and p.Arg384Gln exert their effect on hydroxylation by impairing hydrogen bonding to the haem moiety; a p.Thr318Met change is thought to affect proton transfer to the bound oxygen molecule, while p.Phe79Ile may lead to alteration in orientation of the protein in the mitochondrial membrane. At least one gene deletion has been described that presumably arose from recombination with *CYP11B2* (the reciprocal event of that seen in GRA), but in the case of 11-hydroxylase deficiency, the 5′ end of the gene, exons 1–4, was encoded by *CYP11B2* and the 3′ end of the hybrid, intron 4-exon 9, by *CYP11B1*. This chimaera still has the ability to express 11-hydroxylase activity but only in the zona glomerulosa and is therefore ineffective in cortisol biosynthesis. Uniparental disomy has also been described where the mutation was only paternal in origin with no maternal contribution. This situation may have arisen either where the paternal chromosome had been replicated in a zygote fertilised by a nullisomic oocyte or where the maternal chromosome was lost from a trisomic zygote.

Once the disorder has been confirmed by genetic testing, it simplifies additional testing of other family members to uncover cryptic disease or to provide prenatal diagnosis.

5.4 Diagnosis

Neonatal: Presentation in the newborn is typically of a full-term baby with ambiguous genitalia indicating either in utero androgen excess or deficiency depending on the sex of the baby. Thus, a karyotype is an essential early test to determine the genetic sex and to assist in the differential diagnosis. In addition, the potential risk of a life-threatening adrenal crisis needs to be considered if a salt-losing form of CAH is present. Initial investigations would therefore include serum electrolytes, cortisol and 17-hydroxyprogesterone, the latter because 21-hydroxylase is the most common cause of virilising CAH. Ideally 17-hydroxyprogesterone should not be analysed by immunoassay because of the interference by fetal adrenal steroids leading to false-positive results. Elevated values, usually less than 20 nmol/L, may be found in CYP11B1 deficiency presumably because of accumulation of 17-hydroxyprogesterone prior to the block (see case study). Serum electrolytes are generally normal in CYP11B1 deficiency although salt-losing crises have been reported so should not be assumed to exclude the diagnosis.

Exclusion of 21-hydroxylase deficiency in a child with an impaired cortisol response to ACTH stimulation would then prompt further investigations for other forms of CAH. Measurement of serum 11-deoxycortisol (compound S) on the basal and stimulated sample may be possible. The cut-off for diagnosis is difficult to define as it needs to exclude carriers, who have only a single defective gene, and the acutely sick. Some genetically confirmed carriers have shown responses of

11-deoxycortisol of up to 39 nmol/L following ACTH although others have shown no difference to controls (less than 9 nmol/L). A post-ACTH value of 11-deoxycortisol five times the upper limit of normal has been proposed for diagnosis. In our experience, patients with 11-hydroxylase deficiency typically have values of 11-deoxycortisol greater than 100 nmol/L on ACTH stimulation.

A urine sample should be taken for steroid profile after 3 days of life and ideally prior to commencement of any treatment. This profile will be useful for all forms of CAH and in the case of 11-hydroxylase deficiency will show the metabolites of 11-deoxycortisol. The prominent neonatal metabolite is 6-hydroxytetrahydro-11-deoxycortisol (6-hydroxyTHS) in the glucuronide fraction along with tetrahydro-11-deoxycortisol (THS). At least one case has been described in the literature where THS was not evident until 2–3 weeks after birth, so the diagnosis of 11-hydroxylase deficiency may require a repeat urine sample.

For those patients presenting later in life with either virilisation or hypertension, a steroid profile is again an integrated test allowing review of a number of different disorders in one urine sample. Serum cortisol, as assessed by ACTH stimulation, is usually significantly impaired and serum 11-deoxycortisol elevated to greater than 100 nmol/L. The urine steroid profile shows excess THS and the hexahydroTHS metabolites along with a reduction of cortisol metabolites depending on the severity of the enzyme deficiency. THS excretion is typically over 1500 ug/24 h and in some cases as high as 80,000 ug/24 h, that is, 30–600 times normal. It has been proposed that calculation of the ratio of THS to cortisol metabolites, that is, THS/(THE + THF + 5aTHF), provides improved specificity over the absolute amount of THS although this will be impacted by concomitant treatment. The 95th centile for this ratio in a control group was reported to be 0.26, with patients significantly higher. Tetrahydrodeoxycorticosterone (THDOC) may also be visible in some profiles but not all as its concentration can be much lower than THS as it is additionally excreted in the bile. Adrenal androgen metabolites (androsterone and aetiocholanolone) may not be initially increased if the underlying mutation has residual 11-hydroxylase activity, but these metabolites are likely to increase with age if untreated, reflecting the increase of androgen precursors produced in this disorder.

Carriers for the disease do not show any significant increase in THS and cortisol metabolites are within normal limits.

The finding of elevated THS and metabolites does not automatically confer a diagnosis of 11-hydroxylase deficiency as these are also produced in excess in some adrenal tumours and in response to treatment by metyrapone (an 11β-hydroxylase inhibitor used for the treatment of Cushing's syndrome), etomidate and some of the antifungal drugs that are cytochrome P450 inhibitors, for example, ketoconazole, fluconazole and posaconazole. In the case of adrenal tumours, virilisation may also be the presenting symptom, but one would not expect a reduction of cortisol metabolites as in 11-hydroxylase deficiency. Any interpretation needs to take these possibilities into account and thus can be aided by clinical details provided with the sample or following discussion with the referring clinician.

5.5 Case Study

5.5.1 Neonatal presentation

A male infant with a family history of 11-hydroxylase deficiency was screened for the disease in the first week of life. A serum 17-hydroxyprogesterone of 12.8 nmol/L was obtained on day 4 (normal <5) that probably reflects accumulation of precursors prior to the block as it was measured with a specific method and not by immunoassay that is prone to non-specific interference.

The urine steroid profile on day 5 showed the characteristic increase in THS and the major neonatal metabolite, 6-hydroxy-THS with minimal amounts of the neonatal cortisol metabolites, tetrahydrocortisone and 6-hydroxytetrahydrocortisone (Fig. 5.3).

Genetic confirmation of the disease was obtained by identification of homozygosity for the familial mutation.

5.5.2 Later Presentation

A male infant presented with virilisation aged 18 months and was assumed to have 21-hydroxylase deficiency. He was treated with glucocorticoid replacement with no confirmatory biochemical investigations recorded. The family subsequently moved to the UK where, at age 11 years, he presented with hypertension (220/140 mmHg) causing retinopathy and cardiomyopathy. Pubertal development was complete (Tanner stage 4 genitalia), and he was at near final height. He was found to have an impaired cortisol response to ACTH stimulation (Table 5.1). In view of the hypertension, 11-deoxycortisol was also measured on the basal sample (Table 5.1) and was found to be markedly elevated.

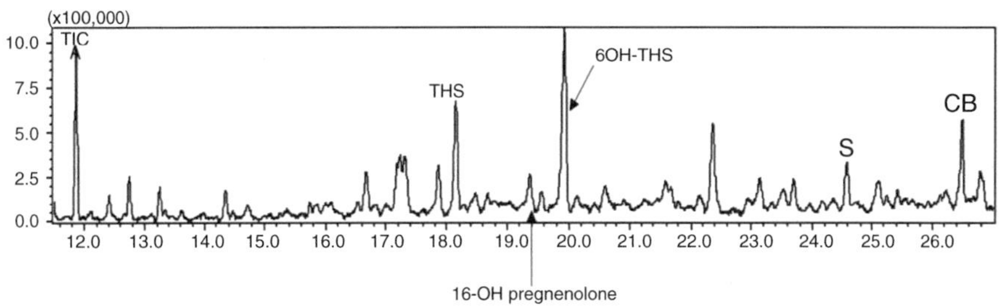

Fig. 5.3 Steroid profile (glucuronide fraction) from a neonate with CYP11B1 deficiency showing dominant 6-hydroxyTHS and THS peaks. A, S and CB are the internal standards. No neonatal cortisol metabolites were found in this spectrum

Table 5.1 Results of ACTH stimulation test

Time	Cortisol (nmol/L)	11-Deoxycortisol (nmol/L)
0	160	>997
30 min	175	Not done

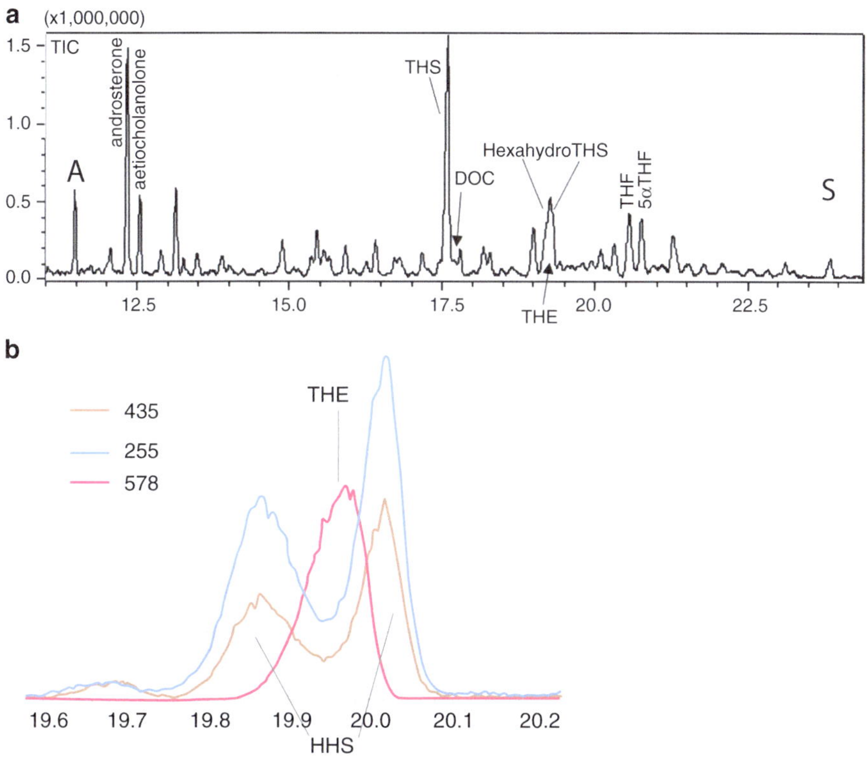

Fig. 5.4 (**a**) Steroid profile from a patient with CYP11B1 deficiency showing markedly decreased cortisol metabolites increased excretion of the adrenal androgens, androsterone and aetiocholanolone, and the presence of excessive amounts of THS and its hexahydro metabolites. DOC is found on the trailing edge of THS. (**b**) Selective ion monitoring of hexahydroTHS (435, 255) and THE (578) showing the overlapping peaks

A urine steroid profile from this patient showed excess THS and HHS metabolites with reduced cortisol metabolites (Fig. 5.4) confirming a diagnosis of 11-hydroxylase deficiency.

Initiation of treatment prior to taking the urine sample may lead to a false-negative result as suppression of ACTH by glucocorticoid replacement will suppress abnormal metabolites and increase cortisol metabolite excretion.

5.6 Steroid Profile

The characteristic metabolites found in urine along with their retention times in terms of methylene units are given in Table 5.2.

In the neonate, 6-hydroxyTHS accounts for approximately 40% of the 11-deoxycortisol metabolites in the first month of life, reflecting the high

Table 5.2 Steroid metabolites relevant to CYP11B1 deficiency, retention times (methylene units, MU) of their MO-TMS derivatives and significant ions (see appendix for spectra)

Steroid	Trivial name	MU	Relevant ions
5β-Pregnan-3α, 6, 17, 21-tetrol-20-one (neonatal metabolite)	6-HydroxyTHS	29.38	652, 562
5β-Pregnan-3α,17, 21-triol-20-one	THS	28.62	564, 474
5β-Pregnan-3α,21-diol-20-one	THDOC	28.64	507, 476
5β-Pregnan-3α,17,20α,21-tetrol	20α HexahydroTHS	29.54	435, 255
5β-Pregnan-3α,17,20β,21-tetrol	20β HexahydroTHS	29.55	435, 255

6α-hydroxylase activity in the neonate. This metabolite elutes just after the 16-hydroxypregnenolone peak (Fig. 5.3). THS itself may not be visible in unfractionated urine containing the neonatal sulphates and glucuronides because it can be obscured by the more abundant 16α,18-dihydroxyDHEA, a product of the fetal adrenal zone. This situation may account for the reported failure to detect THS in the first 2 weeks in some cases of CYP11B1 deficiency. Analysis of the glucuronide fraction separately can clarify the situation. Alternatively, selective ion monitoring for *m*/*z* 595 (the molecular ion of the methyloxime trimethylsilyl derivative of THS) and 564 (formed by loss of the C-20 oxime in this compound) can be used. The hexahydroTHS metabolites of THS are rarely seen at this age.

Later presenting cases will not have the 6-hydroxyTHS metabolite but THS and the hexahydro forms of THS will be present, the latter flanking the tetrahydrocortisone (THE) peak (Fig. 5.4). The tetrahydro metabolite of deoxycorticosterone (THDOC) elutes at the tail end of THS and has been reported to be greater than 3000 ug/24 h in one patient with CYP11B1 deficiency, falling to 140 ug/24 h on treatment, but this is not reflected in the size of the peak on the steroid profile. The adrenal androgens, androsterone and aetiocholanolone, are elevated reflecting the redirection of steroids down the adrenal androgen pathway, while cortisol metabolites may be absent or significantly reduced.

5.6.1 Drug Inhibition of CYP11B1

As previously mentioned, the antifungal azole drugs can inhibit CYP11B1 to various degrees. In our experience, posaconazole and fluconazole can both lead to significant elevations of THS and HHS. One patient with Hodgkin's lymphoma was found to have THS excretion of 2240 ug/24 h (normal <180). As clinical and medication information is frequently lacking, the presence of normal amounts of cortisol metabolites would lead one to question a diagnosis of CYP11B1 in such cases unless of course hydrocortisone replacement had commenced.

5.7 Treatment

As with other forms of CAH treatment, CYP11B1 deficiency requires glucocorticoid replacement to suppress the ACTH drive. Titration of treatment to simulate the diurnal rhythm of cortisol production is difficult as it needs to also suppress adrenal androgen synthesis. No mineralocorticoid replacement is required although for those patients with long-standing hypertension, additional antihypertensive medication may be required.

Further Reading

Clinical Diagnosis and Management

Bulsari K, Falhammer H. Clinical perspectives in congenital adrenal hyperplasia due to 11β-hydroxylase deficiency. Endocrine. 2017;55(1):19–36.

Khattab A, Haider S, Kumar A, et al. Clinical, genetic, and structural basis of congenital adrenal hyperplasia due to 11β-hydroxylase deficiency. Proc Natl Acad Sci U S A. 2017;114(10):E1933–40.

3β-Hydroxysteroid Dehydrogenase/Isomerase Deficiency

6

Gill Rumsby

6.1 Introduction

The 3β-hydroxysteroid dehydrogenase/isomerase (3βHSD) enzyme catalyses the dehydrogenation of the hydroxyl group at carbon 3 of the steroid molecule to a ketone as well as isomerisation of the double bond in the steroid B ring, between carbons 5 and 6, to the A ring carbons 4 and 5 (Fig. 6.1). Thus, the enzyme plays a key role in the conversion of the delta 5 (Δ5) to the delta 4 (Δ4) steroids and is therefore essential for the synthesis of mineralocorticoids, glucocorticoids and androgens.

The enzyme reaction catalysed by 3βHSD requires the presence of the cofactor NAD^+ that is subsequently reduced to NADH. Prior to release of the cofactor from the active site, isomerisation to the Δ4 steroid is carried out in a reaction that appears to be activated by NADH. The enzyme has a similar catalytic efficiency with a variety of substrates and can convert pregnenolone to progesterone, 17-hydroxypregnenolone to 17-hydroxyprogesterone (17OHP), dehydroepiandrosterone (DHEA) to androstenedione and androstenediol to testosterone. It will therefore compete with the 17-hydroxylase enzyme for the metabolism of pregnenolone and 17-hydroxypregnenolone and with the DHEA-sulphotransferase enzyme, SULT2A1, for DHEA.

There are two 3βHSD isoenzymes, type 1 (3βHSD1) and type 2 (3βHSD2); both are microsomal and both use NAD^+ as a cofactor. They do, however, differ in their tissue distribution with 3βHSD2 expressed in the steroid-producing tissues of the adrenal, ovary and testes and 3βHSD1 in placenta and peripheral tissues including the liver, prostate and skin.

G. Rumsby
Department of Clinical Biochemistry, University College London Hospitals, London, UK
e-mail: gill.rumsby@nhs.net

G. Rumsby, G. M. Woodward (eds.), *Disorders of Steroidogenesis*,
https://doi.org/10.1007/978-3-319-96364-8_6

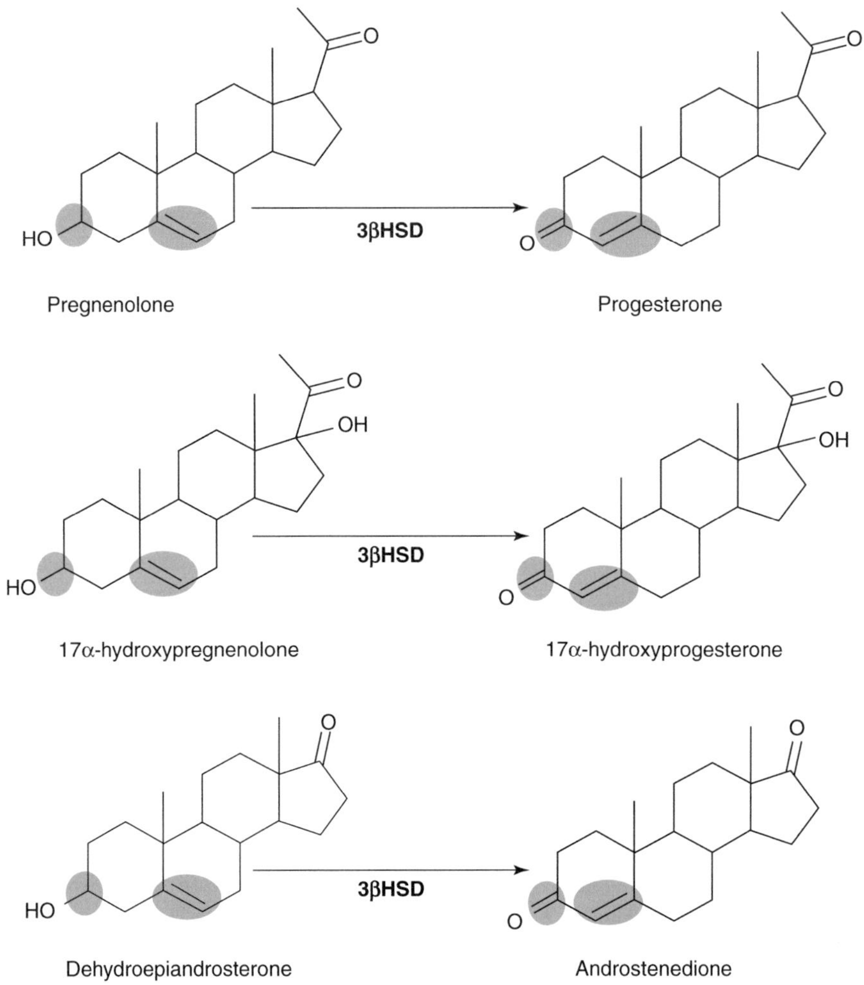

Fig. 6.1 The enzyme 3βHSD2 catalyses the conversion of the Δ5 to Δ4 steroids and also the dehydrogenation of the hydroxyl group at carbon 3, converting pregnenolone to progesterone, 17-hydroxypregnenolone to 17-hydroxyprogesterone and DHEA to androstenedione

The enzyme is poorly expressed in the fetal zone of the fetal adrenal gland but is seen in the neocortex and transitional zones from 24 weeks' gestation. Thus, the fetal adrenal produces large amounts of DHEA and DHEA-sulphate and leads to the characteristic neonatal urine steroid profile consisting of a high output of sulphated Δ5 steroids (see Chaps. 1 and 3). As the fetal adrenal involutes, one sees an increase in delta 4 steroid production in the zona glomerulosa and fasciculata. The zona reticularis, the inner zone of the adrenal, remains relatively deficient in 3βHSD activity as it develops, and this remains low throughout adulthood in contrast to strong expression in the fasciculata and glomerulosa. The mechanism(s) behind this transcriptional regulation is as yet unknown. Thus the main product of the zona reticularis is DHEA-sulphate and the marked increase in production of this steroid around 8 years of age is known as adrenarche.

Deficiency of 3βHSD activity is an underlying cause of one of the rarer, salt-losing forms of congenital adrenal hyperplasia (CAH). The disorder predominantly leads to a 46XY disorder of sex development (DSD), with lack of virilisation in the male infant ranging from perineal hypospadias through to female external genitalia. Females, however, can have some degree of virilisation including clitoromegaly, thus deficiency can be a cause of both 46XX and 46XY DSD. Aldosterone deficiency can lead to a salt-losing crisis that may be fatal in the newborn. Non-salt-losing forms of the disease have been described that may reflect differences in severity of mutations.

The activity of the other isoenzyme, 3βHSD1 can lead to diagnostic confusion as some 17-hydroxyprogesterone may be synthesised although not to the degree seen in 21-hydroxylase deficiency. This additional enzyme activity may also contribute to virilisation in the female as testosterone can be produced in peripheral tissues.

6.2 Presentation

The majority of patients present in the neonatal period with a salt-losing crisis characterised by excessive weight loss, nausea and vomiting or floppiness. These symptoms arise as a result of impaired aldosterone synthesis and can be life threatening. Genital ambiguity, particularly perineal hypospadias in male newborns, may be the first indication that something is amiss, and a karyotype is an essential requirement to establish whether the child is a virilised female or under-virilised male.

Presentation outside the neonatal period may be with either salt-wasting, sometimes precipitated by infection, or because of excess androgen production in females leading to premature puberty. Late-presenting disease is thought to reflect mutations with less severe effects on enzyme function.

6.3 Genetics

Both 3βHSD isoenzymes are encoded by genes located on the short arm of chromosome 1 at 1p13.1. The type 2 enzyme, encoded by *HSD3B2*, shares approximately 93% amino acid sequence similarity with the type 1, 3βHSD1. The *HSD3B2* gene is composed of four exons; the first is non-coding, and the fourth is quite large encoding amino acids 103–372, the bulk of the protein. A variety of mutations have been described in the gene; the majority of these are missense changes, but there are also deletions, frameshift mutations and splice mutations. In some cases, for example, the amino acid change from a glycine to aspartate at amino acid 15 (p.Gly15Asp), the change occurs in the cofactor-binding domain. Thus, the mutated protein may demonstrate some residual enzyme activity in vitro when excessive amounts of the cofactor NAD^+ can be added, whereas the phenotypic appearance of the patient may suggest complete enzyme deficiency. In others, for example, p.Lys173Arg, the enzyme has approximately 50% of normal activity in vitro but is unstable.

Genetic testing is invaluable for diagnosis of other family members and for prenatal diagnosis.

6.4 Diagnosis

In common with other forms of CAH, one of the early diagnostic tests is karyotype analysis to establish whether the child is a virilised female or under-virilised male, and this confirmation can be helpful in pursuing a differential diagnosis. The differential diagnosis of a salt-losing presentation would include 21-hydroxylase, 3βHSD and possibly 11-hydroxylase deficiencies along with disorders in the early part of the steroid pathway as well as renal tubular defects. Depending on the chromosomal sex of the child, this differential can then be narrowed down depending on whether androgen excess (virilised female) or deficiency (partially virilised male) is suspected. Serum electrolytes, cortisol and 17-hydroxyprogesterone should be measured, the hormones ideally by specific methodologies, for example, LCMS, as there can be interference from neonatal steroids in immunoassays. In addition, an ACTH stimulation test should be performed with measurement of cortisol and 17-hydroxyprogesterone pre and post ACTH to confirm that adrenal function is impaired and to exclude 21-hydroxylase deficiency. 17-Hydroxyprogesterone may be slightly elevated in 3βHSD deficiency as a result of 3βHSD type 1 activity, although usually less than 50 nmol/L. A urine sample should be taken after day 3, ideally prior to treatment, and provides the best means of diagnosis of any of the steroid defects providing an overview of all the metabolic pathways affected (Fig. 6.2). The urine profile from a neonate with 3βHSD deficiency is characterised

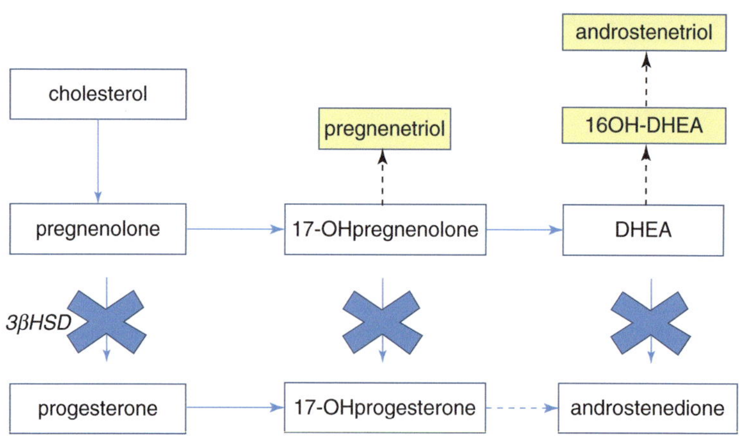

Fig. 6.2 Illustration of the metabolic block caused by 3βHSD2 deficiency with the major urinary steroid metabolites highlighted in yellow

Table 6.1 Hormone levels post ACTH stimulation for exclusion of 3βHSD

	17-Hydroxypregnenolone nmol/L	17-Hydroxypregnenolone/cortisol (nmol/L:nmol/L)
Children premature puberty	<72	<0.067
Adults (hirsute females)	<150	<0.151

by an excess of Δ5 metabolites, but this can also occur if the baby is premature so a degree of caution is required in interpreting these results.

Outside the neonatal period, following confirmation of impaired cortisol synthesis by ACTH stimulation, a urine steroid profile is the most useful test for diagnosis. In untreated patients, there will be excessive amounts of Δ5 steroids produced, particularly DHEA and pregnenetriol (Δ5P3, 5-pregnene-3β,17α,20α-triol), a metabolite of 17-hydroxypregnenolone. This pattern is very similar to that seen in some adrenal tumours that are characterised by an acquired loss of 3βHSD activity (see Chap. 15). One may expect cortisol metabolites to be reduced in inherited 3βHSD deficiency, but nevertheless in the case of mutations that do not fully inactivate the enzyme, these metabolites may still be within the reference range albeit at the low end. Genetic testing is helpful to confirm the diagnosis. Milder degrees of enzyme deficiency have been proposed as the underlying cause of hirsutism, premature sexual hair growth and menstrual disorders in a large number of cases based on basal and stimulated serum 17-hydroxypregnenolone and DHEA concentrations and the ratio of these steroids to the Δ4 steroids 17-hydroxyprogesterone and androstenedione, respectively. These diagnoses appeared excessive in terms of the expected incidence of the disease and have not subsequently been borne out by genetic testing. The poor discrimination of Δ5 to Δ4 ratio of serum steroid results with and without ACTH stimulation has been suggested to be the result of the influence of 3βHSD type 1. Hormonal criteria for diagnosis using 17-hydroxypregnenolone and 17-hydroxypregnenolone to cortisol ratio have been proposed based on comparison of genetically proven cases with those from other high-risk groups (Table 6.1). In all cases, 17-hydroxypregnenolone was greater than 100 nmol/L post ACTH stimulation.

6.5 Case Study

A baby born at full term with normal delivery was found on routine examination to have perineal hypospadias and a small penis. The gonads were impalpable but shown on ultrasound to be present in the inguinal canals.

Serum biochemistry on day 2 showed a testosterone of 15 nmol/L, 17-hydroxyprogesterone 40 nmol/L (<5) with LH and FSH both <0.1 IU/L. Cortisol response to Synacthen was impaired: 110 nmol/L (basal) and 109 nmol/L at 60 min confirming adrenal insufficiency. A urine sample was taken for steroid profile analysis, and the child was discharged on hydrocortisone replacement. Subsequent karyotype analysis confirmed a 46XY genotype.

He was readmitted on day 5 in a salt-losing crisis: vomiting and dehydrated. Serum sodium was 108 mmol/L, potassium 7.1 mmol/L and urea 12 mmol/L. A urine sample was also taken at this time.

The differential diagnosis is of a salt-losing form of congenital adrenal hyperplasia. While the testosterone suggests that a virilising form of CAH is present, serum 17-hydroxyprogesterone, taken pretreatment, is not high enough to suggest that the underlying cause is 21-hydroxylase deficiency, the most common form of CAH. The other possibilities that need to be considered are 11-hydroxylase deficiency, more usually associated with hypertension but can present with salt-losing in early life, or 3βHSD deficiency where the other peripheral isoenzyme can metabolise some of the Δ5 precursors to 17-hydroxyprogesterone. Earlier defects in the pathway, for example, cholesterol side chain cleavage and steroidogenic acute regulatory protein deficiency, are excluded because of the presence of significant amounts of testosterone and 17-hydroxyprogesterone.

The steroid profile showed almost undetectable neonatal cortisol metabolites and the characteristic high Δ5 steroid metabolites, DHEA, androstenetriol (androst-5-ene-16α,17β-triol), 16-hydroxypregnenolone and Δ5P3 suggestive of a diagnosis of 3βHSD deficiency (Fig. 6.3). However, caution does need to be exercised as prematurity can lead to a similar picture of increased Δ5 steroids, and therefore additional confirmation, for example, repeating the urine steroid profile after 1 month post-term to see if levels of the Δ5 metabolites persist, is required, but note that this may be obscured by concurrent treatment. Genetic testing is therefore advisable to confirm the biochemistry.

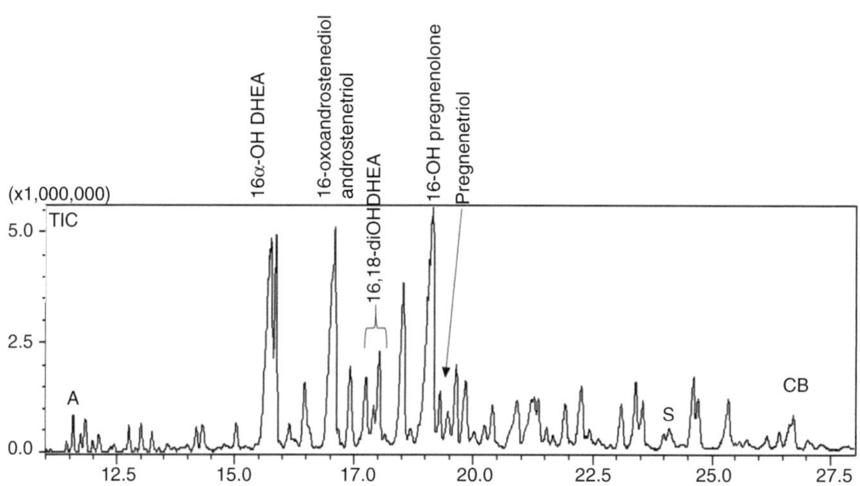

Fig. 6.3 Sulphate fraction from a 21-day-old child subsequently shown to have 3β-HSD deficiency. Note the extremely high excretion of Δ5 steroid metabolites. At this age it can be a difficult disorder to diagnose as the profile bears considerable similarity to that seen prematurity. In this case, no neonatal cortisol metabolites were seen in the glucuronide fraction supporting the diagnosis

In this particular case genetic testing confirmed the diagnosis finding a deleterious change in *HSD3B2*, a duplication, g.5554dupT, leading to a frame shift mutation, p.Leu22Phefs*, that would lead to premature termination and either destruction of the mRNA or synthesis of a truncated form of the protein.

6.6 Steroid Profile

In the neonate the characteristic profile of excess fetal adrenal steroids that are predominantly Δ5 steroids can make diagnosis of 3βHSD deficiency difficult, particularly if the child is premature, as fetal adrenal steroids can persist for several months in the premature infant. In practice the amount of Δ5 steroids, in particular the characteristic neonatal metabolites, 16-hydroxypregnenolone and 16α-hydroxyDHEA (3β,16α-dihydroxy-androst-5-en-17-one), 16β-hydroxyDHEA (3β,16β-dihydroxy-androst-5-en-17-one) and androstenetriol, tend to be extremely high and do not fall with age post-term as one would expect in the normal neonate (Fig. 6.3). It is notable that significant Δ4 steroids may also be present, including pregnanetriol and 17-hydroxypregnanolone (metabolites of 17-hydroxyprogesterone), reflecting the activity of 3βHSD1, and these may lead to a false impression of 21-hydroxylase deficiency. The finding of pregnenediol (derived from pregnenolone) and Δ5P3 adds further support to the diagnosis of 3βHSD deficiency. Δ5Pe is a minor marker in the neonate when compared to the older child/adult with 3βHSD deficiency, but its presence is still useful. The concentration of these metabolites will, however, obviously be reduced by any cortisol replacement regime, and it is vital that the laboratory is notified of the timing of the sample relative to any treatment.

Outside the neonatal period, the diagnosis is less prone to error as there is no contribution from the fetal adrenal to add confusion. Excess DHEA, 16α-hydroxy-DHEA (present as a doublet reflecting the *syn*- and *anti*-forms of the oxime derivative), pregnenediol (5-pregnene 3β,20α-diol) and Δ5P3 are found. It is notable that significant Δ4 steroids are also present, for example, pregnanetriol—a metabolite of 17-hydroxyprogesterone, reflecting the activity of 3βHSD1 (Fig. 6.4). This pattern can also be found in the presence of an adrenal tumour where the tumour tissue becomes relatively 3βHSD deficient (Chap. 15). The mode of presentation would need to be taken into consideration, for example, a sudden onset of virilisation is more likely to indicate a tumour.

A list of typical metabolites and their retention indices (methylene units) is given in Table 6.2.

6.6.1 Inhibitors of 3βHSD

Medroxyprogesterone, a commonly used progestogen, has been demonstrated to inhibit 3βHSD2 in vitro at concentrations that may be physiologically significant. Other inhibitors, such as trilostane used in the treatment of Cushing's syndrome and

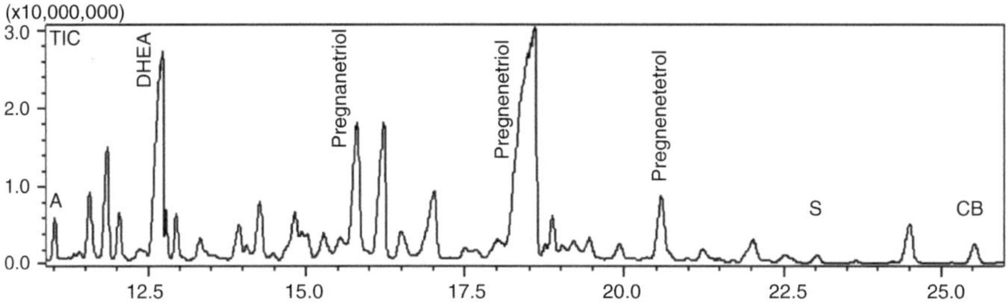

Fig. 6.4 Urine steroid profile from a 3-year-old with 3βHSD2 deficiency. Cortisol metabolites, THE, THF and 5αTHF can only be detected by selective ion monitoring. A, S and CB are the internal standards

Table 6.2 Metabolites seen in 3βHSD2 deficiency, retention times (methylene units, MU) of their MO-TMS derivatives and their characteristic ions (See appendix for spectra)

Steroid	Trivial name	MU	Characteristic ions
5-Androsten-3β-ol-17-one	DHEA	25.75	268, 358
5β-Pregnan-3α,17-diol-20-one	17-Hydroxypregnanolone	27.08	476, 188
5-Androsten-3β,16β-diol-17-one	16-HydroxyDHEA	27.74	266, 446
5β-Pregnan-3α,17,20α-triol	Pregnanetriol	28.00	255, 435
5-Androsten-3β,17β-diol-16-one 5-Androsten-3β,15β,16α-triol-17-one	16-Oxoandrostenediol and 15β,16α-dihydroxyDHEA[a]	28.20	446, 356 565, 232
5-Androsten-3β,16β,17β-triol	Androstenetriol	28.45	432, 329
5-Androsten-3β,16α,18-triol-17-one	16,18-DihydroxyDHEA[a]	28.65/28.81	388, 283
5-Pregnen-3β,16α-diol-20-one	16-Hydroxypregnenolone[a]	29.34	474, 384
5-Pregnen-3β,17α,20α-triol	Pregnenetriol (Δ5P3)	29.42	433, 253
5-Pregnen-3β,15β,17α,20-tetrol		29.80	521, 431, 269

[a]Predominantly neonatal metabolites

its derivative epostane, appear to have a greater affinity for the type 1 enzyme so should not lead to diagnostic confusion.

6.7 Treatment

The mainstay of treatment for 3βHSD deficiency, as for other forms of salt-losing congenital adrenal hyperplasia, is that of replacement with glucocorticoid and mineralocorticoid. Corrective surgery may be required in both males and females and in the former additional androgen.

Further Reading

Diagnosis

Lutfallah C, Wang W, Mason I, Chang YT, et al. Newly proposed hormonal criteria via genotypic proof for type II 3β-hydroxysteroid dehydrogenase deficiency. J Clin Endocrinol Metab. 2002;87:2611–22.

Steroid Profiling

Wolthers BG, de Vries IJ, Volmer M, Nagel GT. Detection of 3β-hydroxysteroid dehydrogenase deficiency in a newborn by means of urinary steroid analysis. Clin Chim Acta. 1987;169:109–16.

17α-Hydroxylase Deficiency

7

Gill Rumsby

7.1 Introduction

The 17α-hydroxylase/17,20-lyase (CYP17) enzyme is a member of the cytochrome P450 group of mixed function oxidases. The enzyme is found in the endoplasmic reticulum of the zona fasciculata and reticularis of the adrenal cortex but not the zona glomerulosa, consistent with its role in androgen and cortisol biosynthesis. CYP17 is also present in gonadal tissues, and consequently enzyme deficiency affects both adrenal and gonadal steroid biosynthesis.

This cytosolic enzyme catalyses two main functions: firstly, hydroxylation at the C17 position of the steroid molecule, an essential step for cortisol biosynthesis, and secondly cleavage of the side chain between C17 and C20 yielding the C19 steroids—the precursors of androgens and oestrogens (Fig. 7.1). The human enzyme favours the delta-5 steroid (Δ5), 17-hydroxypregnenolone, for this step, 17-hydroxyprogesterone being a much poorer substrate with a rate of conversion approximately 3% that of the Δ5 steroid. Consequently, the major adrenal androgen produced is dehydroepiandrosterone (DHEA) and its metabolites. The cleavage of the side chain, converting the C21 steroids to the C19, 17-oxo steroids, occurs primarily in the zona reticularis, the 17-hydroxylation reaction and hence glucocorticoid synthesis, predominating in the zona fasciculata. CYP17 requires molecular oxygen and two electrons for the hydroxylation reaction, the latter provided by NADPH via cytochrome P450 oxidoreductase (POR) to CYP17. The regulation of side chain cleavage is still not clear. From histological studies on the fetal and adult adrenal glands, it is apparent that there is little change in CYP17 expression with age but there are dramatic changes in expression of cytochrome b_5 throughout life. This haemoprotein is an allosteric effector for CYP17 that enhances 17,20-lyase

G. Rumsby
Department of Clinical Biochemistry, University College London Hospitals, London, UK
e-mail: gill.rumsby@nhs.net

G. Rumsby, G. M. Woodward (eds.), *Disorders of Steroidogenesis*,
https://doi.org/10.1007/978-3-319-96364-8_7

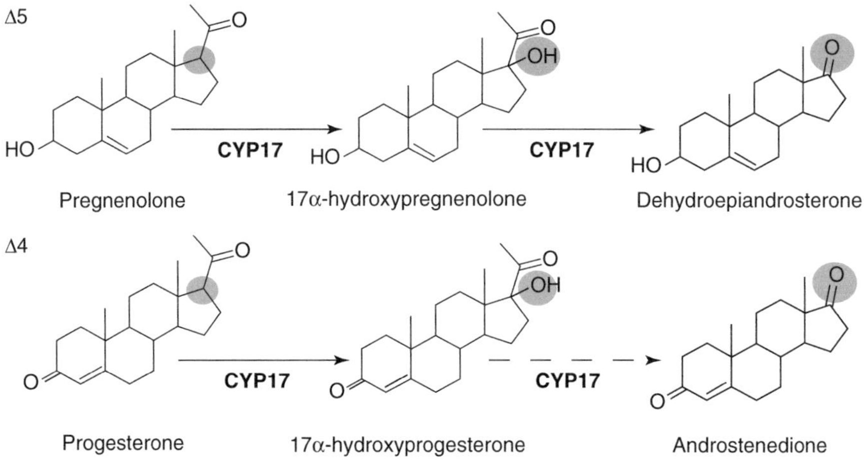

Fig. 7.1 Reactions catalysed by the 17α hydroxylase/17,20-lyase enzyme, CYP17. After addition of the hydroxyl group at C17, the side chain is cleaved between carbons 17 and 20 to yield the C19 steroids. The Δ4 steroid 17-hydroxyprogesterone is a much poorer substrate for the enzyme in humans, and therefore the reaction is denoted by a hatched line

activity approximately tenfold. It is expressed throughout gestation in the fetal and transitional zones of the adrenal cortex, the fetal zone producing a high output of DHEA sulphate. The fetal neocortex, the precursor of adult cortical tissue, shows no expression of cytochrome b_5 until after 23 weeks of gestation. Postnatally the fetal zone involutes, and the neocortex and transitional zone expand to form the zona glomerulosa and fasciculata, respectively. The zona reticularis is initially poorly developed but starts to expand around 5–7 years of age and exhibits increasing expression of cytochrome b_5 that plateaus in the mid-teens. Thus adrenarche, the onset of adrenal androgen production, is associated with the development of the zona reticularis and expression of increased amounts of cytochrome b_5. There is a noticeable drop in adrenal androgen production with ageing, in particular of DHEA sulphate, that appears to be due to a reduction in the size of the zona reticularis rather than any decrease in cytochrome b_5 expression. CYP17 also has the ability to catalyse the 16α-hydroxylation of progesterone but not pregnenolone. From cross-species comparison, this ability appears to be related to the presence of an alanine rather than a leucine at residue 105 perhaps influencing the repositioning of the steroid in the active site.

Gonadal steroid synthesis also requires CYP17 and also favours the Δ5 pathway to DHEA. The testicular Leydig cells can carry out all the steps required for testosterone synthesis from cholesterol. By contrast, in the ovary the enzymes are differentially expressed in the granulosa and thecal cells, and thus oestrogen synthesis requires both cell types. The granulosa cells synthesise pregnenolone and progesterone in response to LH stimulation which then diffuse into the neighbouring thecal cells where CYP17 and 3β-hydroxysteroid dehydrogenase metabolise them to androstenedione. The androstenedione then returns to the granulosa cells to act as a substrate for the aromatase enzyme and oestrogen synthesis.

CYP17 has also been implicated in the so-called back door pathway of androgen production in which 17-hydroxyprogesterone is initially metabolised by 5α-reductase and 3α-hydroxysteroid reductase to 17-hydroxy allopregnanolone (5α-pregnan 3α,17β-diol-20-one), a substrate for CYP17 lyase. The androsterone produced is then oxidised at the C3 position to form the active androgen, dihydrotestosterone. The reaction of CYP17 with this substrate is not influenced by cytochrome b5, and the pathway has been suggested to contribute to the virilisation seen in steroid 21-hydroxylase and P450 oxidoreductase (POR) deficiencies in which 17-hydroxyprogesterone accumulates.

CYP17 deficiency is a rare form of congenital adrenal hyperplasia (CAH) accounting for less than 1% of cases. Its phenotype primarily reflects the inability to produce both cortisol and gonadal sex steroids hence a failure of virilisation of the male and pubertal failure and absence of secondary sexual characteristics (no axial or pubic hair, minimal breast development) in the female. Thus, the condition is classified as a disorder of sex development (DSD). Aldosterone is unaffected as the enzyme is not required for its synthesis. The low renin hypertension associated with this disorder is thought to arise because of the synthesis of increased corticosterone precursors either because the excess progesterone is channelled into aldosterone synthesis or from the accumulation of precursors with mineralocorticoid activity, for example, deoxycorticosterone. In cases where enzyme activity is not fully lost, there may be genital ambiguity in the male including various degrees of hypospadias, undescended testes and the presence of inguinal hernia. Some cases have been described where there is selective loss of the lyase reaction but with preserved glucocorticoid production (see Sect. 7.3). Such cases have been invaluable in identifying residues in the CYP17 protein that interact with POR and cytochrome b_5, in some cases leading to the identification of mutations in these other genes.

7.2 Presentation

In the neonate this disorder is most likely to present with genital ambiguity, and the chromosomal sex is essential to establish whether the child is an under-virilised male or a virilised female and hence the direction of further investigations. Inguinal hernias, caused by undescended testes, may be found in the male, and these would point to a failure of androgen synthesis, for whatever reason, as the underlying cause. Genetic females (i.e. 46XX) are unlikely to present at this time.

More typically CYP17 deficiency presents in the teenage years with pubertal failure and symptoms associated with persistent hypertension. Serum progesterone is likely to be elevated and gives a strong clue to the diagnosis. Gonadotropins may also be elevated consistent with primary gonadal failure. Low renin hypertension may also be present and may lead to suppressed aldosterone. On examination, sexual infantilism, minimal breast development and absence of pubic and axillary hair are also typical findings. As in the neonate, a karyotype and urine steroid profile are important tests to aid diagnosis. Genetic males have absent or incomplete development of the external genitalia. Genetic females, that is, 46XX, also have hypertension and hypergonadotrophic hypogonadism along with impaired fertility as a result of follicular arrest although normal menstruation has been reported in some cases.

7.3 Genetics

The *CYP17A1* gene encoding this enzyme is found on chromosome 10q24.3. From naturally occurring mutations, we now know that there are some residues that are important in the interaction with cytochrome b5 and POR (see below). Transcription is restricted to the adrenal and gonads with expression under the influence of several transcription factors including steroidogenic factor 1 (SF1).

More than 50 mutations have been described to date—a mixture of minor deletions and missense changes. As the disease is rare, most mutations are family specific. There are, however, three recurrent mutations described: (1) a deletion of three nucleotides encoding phenylalanine at codon 54 (p.Phe54del) found in patients of Asian and Japanese origin; (2) a duplication of four nucleotides in exon 8 leading to a frameshift mutation, p.Pro480Hisfs*, found in Canadian Mennonites; and (3) a missense change, p.Trp406Arg, that accounts for approximately 50% mutant alleles in Brazilian patients.

Two changes, p.Arg347His and p.Arg358Gln, have been described that predominantly impair the 17,20-lyase function and therefore androgen synthesis, while glucocorticoid synthesis remains intact. These mutations illustrate the role of electrostatic interactions with POR and cytochrome b_5, essential for side chain cleavage to occur.

At least two cases have been described where deficiency of 17,20-lyase activity is not the result of mutation within *CYP17* itself but is caused by a mutation in either POR or cytochrome b_5 affecting their interaction with CYP17. This finding of course has implications for genetic testing and diagnosis of other family members, and thus it is recommended that CYP17 deficiency is confirmed by genotyping of the relevant genes.

7.4 Diagnosis

As previously mentioned, CYP17 deficiency in the neonate is most likely to present with genital ambiguity. One of the first tests must therefore be a karyotype to determine whether the cause is androgen insufficiency or excess. If 46XY, then disorders of androgen synthesis need to be considered including CYP17 deficiency and earlier defects in the cortisol biosynthetic pathway as well as gonadal steroid disorders such as 17β-hydroxysteroid dehydrogenase and 5α-reductase deficiencies and androgen receptor disorders. Serum cortisol and its response to ACTH stimulation should be assessed early to review adrenal function and, in the case of CYP17 deficiency, this will be impaired. A urine steroid profile can then be used to further elucidate the adrenal disorder. If male then further investigation of gonadal steroid function may be required including stimulation of the testes with human chorionic gonadotrophin (hCG), measuring testosterone before and after stimulation. Serum steroids can be ambiguous in the neonate when analysed by immunoassay methods because of non-specific interference from fetal adrenal steroids, and therefore several different tests may be required to confirm the diagnosis. A number of LCMS methods are now available and are generally to be preferred for serum hormone analysis, but even these are not without problems as, depending on the chromatography conditions, there may be overlap with other, isobaric steroids. One pertinent example reported was the finding of an apparently elevated 11-deoxycortisol making a diagnosis of 11β-hydroxylase deficiency in a child subsequently found on urine steroid profile to have 17α-hydroxylase deficiency. This error related to the co-elution of 11-deoxycortisol with the isobaric steroid corticosterone. A longer chromatography separation time was able to resolve the two compounds. A urine steroid profile of the sulphate conjugates in the neonate shows a characteristic pattern of raised metabolites of pregnenolone and decreased DHEA metabolites illustrating the inability to produce C19 steroids.

For patients presenting in later life with either hypertension or pubertal failure, one would expect to see increased serum progesterone reflecting the accumulation of precursors. Median values of 28.7 nmol/L (interquartile range 18–42) have been reported. Cortisol response to ACTH stimulation is typically poor in those with complete deficiency of the enzyme. The urine steroid profile in complete CYP17 deficiency shows increased progesterone metabolites along with increased output of corticosterone metabolites (Figs. 7.2 and 7.3).

7.5 Case Study

7.5.1 Neonatal Presentation

A patient born at full term was noted to have undescended testes, small phallus and penoscrotal hypospadias at birth. The differential diagnosis included disorders of androgen biosynthesis and androgen action: 17α-hydroxylase deficiency, 17β-hydroxysteroid dehydrogenase deficiency, 5α reductase deficiency and androgen receptor defects. Initial tests showed that cortisol response to stimulation was poor, 27 nmol/L rising to 201 nmol/L at 60 min. Serum testosterone showed a minimal response to a 3-week hCG stimulation test rising from 2.6 to 3.3 nmol/L. The karyotype was found to be 46XY. These results indicate impaired androgen and cortisol synthesis suggestive of either CYP17 or 3β-hydroxysteroid dehydrogenase deficiency.

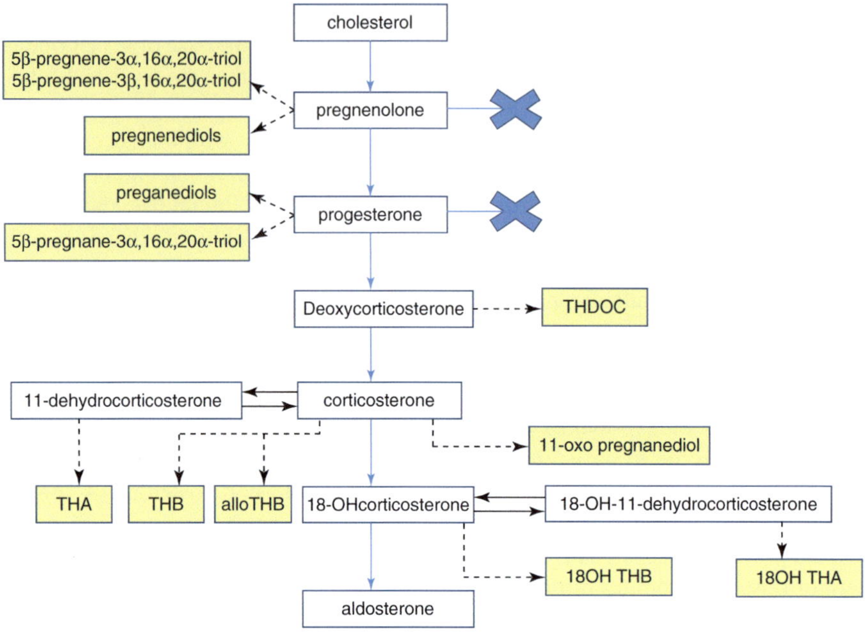

Fig. 7.2 Illustration of the metabolic block caused by CYP17 deficiency and the urinary metabolites produced highlighted in yellow. *THA* tetrahydro-11-dehydrocorticosterone, *THB* tetrahydrocorticosterone, *THDOC* tetrahydrodeoxycorticosterone

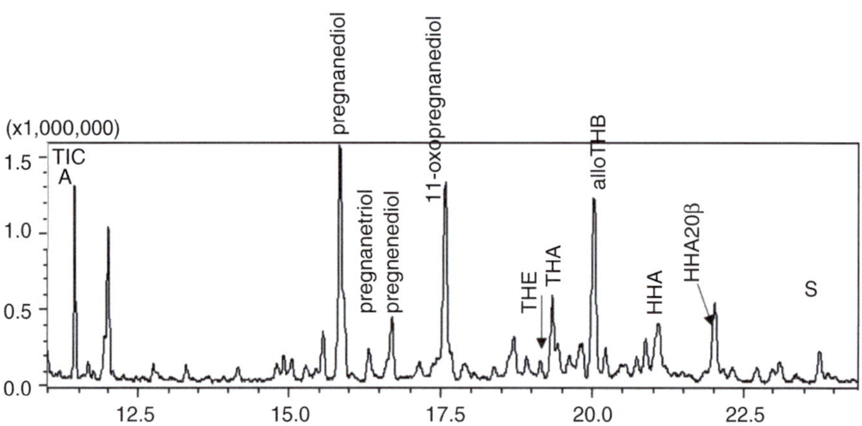

Fig. 7.3 Urine steroid profile from a 15-year-old 46XY female with CYP17 deficiency clearly showing a lack of adrenal androgens and an excess of progesterone, pregnenolone and corticosterone metabolites. A and S denote the internal standards androstanediol and stigmasterol, respectively

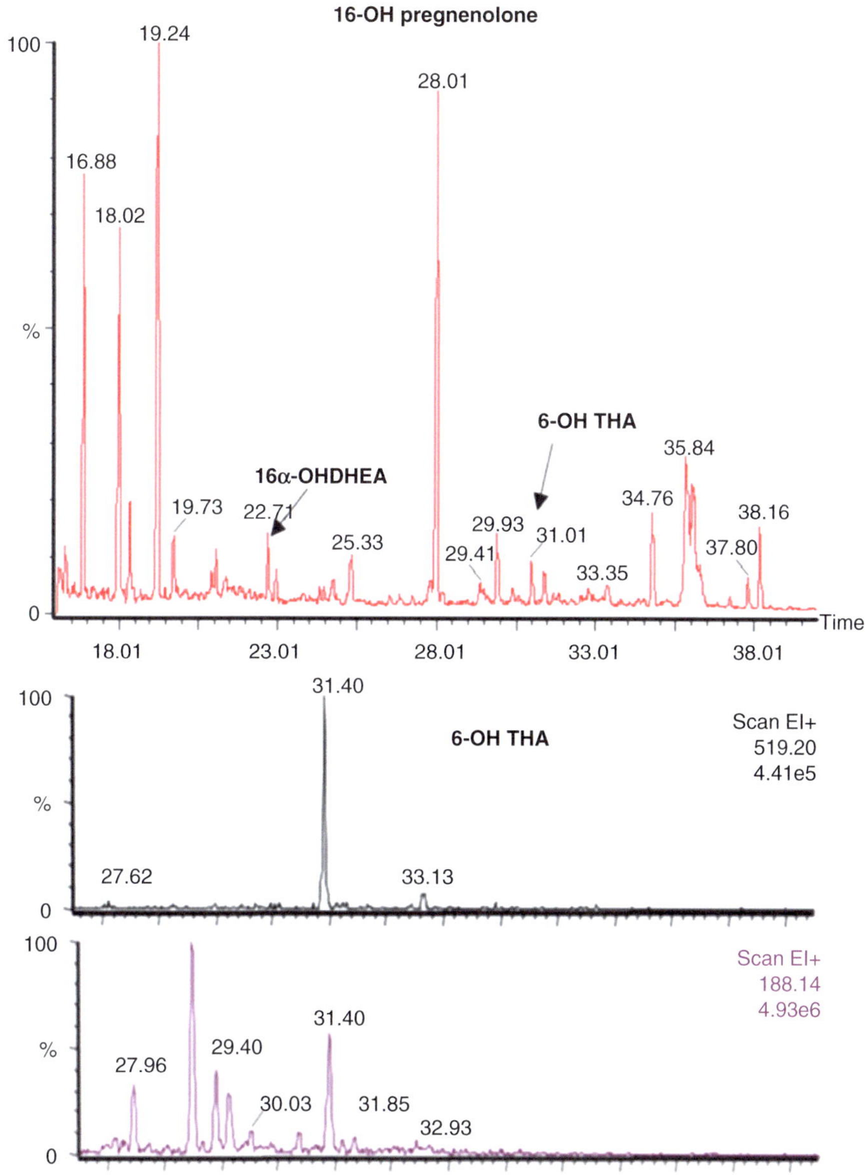

Fig. 7.4 Sulphate fraction from urine steroid profile from neonate with CYP17 deficiency showing the marked increase of 16α-hydroxypregnenolone compared to the C19 metabolite 16α-hydroxyDHEA. The 6OHTHA neonatal metabolite is present in both the sulphate and glucuronide fractions and can be identified by the ions at 519 and 188 (spectrum kindly provided by Dr. N. Taylor)

Analysis of the urine steroid profile showed a dominant peak of 16-hydroxypregnenolone, the neonatal metabolite of pregnenolone with minimal amounts of 16α-hydroxy-dehydroepiandrosterone (16αOHDHEA) and other C19 steroids (Fig. 7.4).

Table 7.1 ACTH stimulation in a 18-year-old female presenting with primary amenorrhoea and pubertal delay

Time post-ACTH stimulation	Cortisol (nmol/L)
0 min	178
60 min	186
Normal response	>550 at 60 min

In the above case, genetic testing identified a homozygous 3-base pair deletion, c.160_162delTTC, that led to deletion of a phenylalanine residue at position 54 in the CYP17 protein. This mutation is known to be pathological leading to a partial loss of 17-hydroxylase enzyme activity and almost complete absence of 17,20-lyase activity in vitro.

7.5.2 Adult Presentation

An 18-year-old female presented for assessment of primary amenorrhoea and pubertal delay. She had normal external genitalia and vaginal appearance. Breast development had commenced at age 15 but only progressed to Tanner stage II. Ovaries were visible on ultrasound and karyotype shown to be 46XX. Her blood pressure ranged from 120/80 to 150/100 mmHg.

Biochemical investigations showed that she had an elevated progesterone of 12 nmol/L (normal <6), undetectable renin and a subnormal response of cortisol to Synacthen stimulation (Table 7.1). The urine steroid profile (Fig. 7.3) was characterised by increased pregnanediol, a progesterone metabolite, along with tetrahydro-11-dehydrocorticosterone (THA) and 5α-tetrahydrocorticosterone (alloTHB), both metabolites of corticosterone. Adrenal androgens were very low.

Whole gene sequencing of *CYP17A1* demonstrated the same c.160_162del (p.Phe54del) homozygous mutation seen in the neonatal case presented above.

7.6 Steroid Profile

Metabolites arise from pregnenolone, progesterone, deoxycorticosterone, corticosterone, 18-hydroxycorticosterone and 18-hydroxydeoxycorticosterone (Fig. 7.2, Table 7.2). In addition, there are some 21-deoxy, 11-oxygenated steroids, for example, 5β-pregnane-3α,11β,20α-triol, derived from the action of bacterial 21-dehydroxylase on corticosterone; the steroids are subsequently reabsorbed from the gut and excreted in the urine.

A urine steroid profile in the neonate with CYP17 deficiency is characterised by raised metabolites of pregnenolone, in particular 16OHPe, and decreased 16αOHDHEA illustrating the inability to produce C19 steroids. The ratio of these two metabolites has been proposed as a useful discriminant for diagnosis in the neonate as it can be around 10- to 20-fold that seen in normal neonates. These metabolites are particularly evident in the sulphate fraction of the profile that is analysed separately from the glucuronide fraction in the first month of life (see Sect. 7.5; Fig. 7.4).

Table 7.2 Steroid metabolites characteristic of CYP17 deficiency, retention times (methylene units, MU) of their MO-TMS derivatives and relevant ions (see appendix for spectra)

Steroid	Trivial name	MU	Relevant ions
5α-Pregnane-3α,20α-diol	5α-Pregnanediol	27.55	117, 269
5-Pregnene-3β,20α-diol	Pregnenediol (5PD)	28.16	117, 372
5β-Pregnane-3α,20α-diol	Pregnanediol (PD)	28.31	117, 269
3α,20α-Dihydroxy-5β-pregnan-11-one	11-Oxopregnanediol	28.66	388, 334
3α,21-Dihydroxy-5β-pregnane-20-one	THDOC	28.93/29.72[a]	476, 188
5-Pregnene-3β, 16α,20α-triol		29.6	460, 445, 117
3α,21-Dihydroxy-5β-pregnane-11,20 dione	THA	29.77	188, 400
5β-Pregnane-3α,11β,21-triol-20-one	THB	30.00/30.16[a]	564, 188
5α-Pregnane-3α,11β,21-triol-20-one	5αTHB	30.16/30.80[a]	474, 188
3α,20α,21-Trihydroxy-5β-pregnan-11-one	HHA	30.76	373, 283
5β-Pregnane- 3α,11β,20α,21-tetrol	HHB	31.15	267, 357
Neonatal metabolites			
5-Androsten-3β,16α-diol-17-one	16αOHDHA	27.38/27.42[a]	266, 446
5-Pregnen-3β,16α-diol-20-one	16-OH preg	29.38	474, 384
6α-Hydroxy tetrahydro-11-dehydrocorticosterone	6OHTHA	30.86/31.52[a]	519, 188

[a]Denotes retention times for *syn*- and *anti*-forms

There is also a predominance of 11-dehydrocorticosterone (THA) metabolites in the neonate, particularly the 6α-hydroxylated form, 6OHTHA. This finding is in marked contrast to the predominance of corticosterone metabolites seen in older children and adults and reflects the high activity of 11β-hydroxysteroid dehydrogenase 2 in the neonate.

By contrast, in older children and adults the major corticosteroid metabolites are those of corticosterone: tetrahydrocorticosterone (THB), 5αTHB, THA and 5αTHA (Fig. 7.3). In addition, there is an excess of metabolites derived from pregnenolone and progesterone: pregnenediol and pregnanediol and the 16-hydroxylated derivatives of these (5-pregnene-3β,16α,20α-triol, 5-pregnene-3α,16α,20α-triol and 5β-pregnan-3α,16α,20α-triol). An 11-hydroxylated form of pregnanetriol can also be produced possibly by the 21-dehydroxylation of THB and 5αTHB. Cortisol metabolites THE, THF and 5αTHF would be expected to be significantly reduced in complete enzyme deficiency as would the adrenal androgens, androsterone (An) and aetiocholanolone (Ae). The ratio of (5PD + PD)/(An + Ae) has been reported to be significantly elevated in CYP17 deficiency, some 4000-8000 times normal, and there is an increase of corticosterone over cortisol metabolites (THB + 5αTHB/THF + 5αTHF + THE).

Tetrahydrodeoxycorticosterone (THDOC), the major metabolite of deoxycorticosterone, is difficult to resolve from 11-oxopregnanediol, a metabolite of 11-hydroxyprogesterone, as the latter is present in considerably higher amounts. Quantitation is therefore difficult unless performed by selective ion monitoring looking for ions at 507 (molecular ion, M^+) and 476 (M-31).

The 18-hydroxy metabolites of THDOC and THB are also present but without an associated increase in aldosterone. It is thought that these metabolites are synthesised in the zona fasciculata from the excess corticosterone produced under the stimulus of ACTH, presumably by the 11-hydroxylase enzyme that has some 18-hydroxylase capability. Aldosterone synthesis in the zona glomerulosa is characteristically reduced in CYP17 deficiency. 18-OHTHDOC can be detected by selective ion monitoring for the molecular ion at m/e 595, 564 (M^{+}-31) and 443 (M^{+}-152).

In those instances where the lyase step is selectively impaired either because of a mutation in *CYP17A1* itself or as the result of mutation in POR or cytochrome b5, cortisol synthesis may be preserved, but abnormal corticosterone metabolites will still be present (see Chap. 14). The ratio of pregnanetriol/(An + Ae) has been reported to be elevated in patients with lyase deficiency (mean of 2.23 compared to 0.2 in controls).

7.6.1 Inhibitors of CYP17

A number of inhibitors of CYP17 have been described including abiraterone, orteronel and TDK-001—orteronel being more specific than the others. Such inhibitors, by reduction of androgen production, have potential benefits for the treatment of prostate cancer, and one of these, abiraterone, has also been proposed as a potential treatment of hyperandrogenism in virilising forms of CAH although glucocorticoid replacement would obviously still be required.

7.7 Treatment

Treatment requires glucocorticoid but not mineralocorticoid replacement. The hypertension typically resolves when glucocorticoid replacement is implemented.

Further Reading

Spectral Details of Metabolites

Honour JW, Tourniaire J, Biglieri EG, Shackleton CHL. Urinary steroid excretion in 17α-hydroxlase deficiency. J Steroid Biochem. 1978;9:495–505.

General

Auchus R. Steroid 17-hydroxylase and 17,20 lyase deficiencies, genetic and pharmacologic. J Steroid Biochem Mol Biol. 2017;165(Pt A:71–8.

Storbeck KH, Swart AC, Fox CL, Swart P. Cytochrome b5 modulates multiple reactions in steroidogenesis by diverse mechanisms. J Steroid Biochem Mol Biol. 2015;151:66–73.

Early Defects of Steroidogenesis: Steroidogenic Acute Regulatory Protein and Cholesterol 20-22 Lyase Deficiency

8

Edmund H. Wilkes and Gary M. Woodward

8.1 Introduction

As described in Chap. 1, steroid hormones are primarily synthesised in the adrenal glands from cholesterol. The transport of cholesterol into adrenal cells, and their intracellular compartments (i.e. the mitochondria), is crucial for the synthesis of steroid hormones. This step is achieved, in part, by the binding of circulating low-density lipoproteins (LDL) to LDL receptors on the surface of adrenal cells and internalisation of LDL by receptor-mediated endocytosis to form endosomes. Cholesterol can also be synthesized *de novo* in the endoplasmic reticulum. This process is described in more detail in Chap. 14. Cholesterol is present within the cell as either free cholesterol or cholesterol esters (produced via the action of acyl-CoA:cholesterol transferase). Free cholesterol, mainly produced by the action of hormone-sensitive lipase, interacts with a number of proteins containing a steroidogenic acute regulatory protein (StAR)-related lipid transfer (START) domain. These proteins have a variety of functions including transcription factors and mediators of cholesterol transport. There are three START domain (StarD) proteins – StarD4, D5 and D6 – which are involved in trans-cytoplasmic transfer of cholesterol to the outer mitochondrial membrane. The StAR protein is found in all steroidogenic tissues, excluding the placenta, and contains an N-terminal targeting sequence that permits its mitochondrial uptake. Once inside the mitochondrion, however, this sequence is cleaved and the protein ceases to mediate cholesterol uptake. Taken together, StAR acts to facilitate the transport of cholesterol from the outer to the inner mitochondrial membrane and to make the substrate available to the cholesterol side-chain cleavage enzyme (CYP11A1) for the first step of steroidogenesis (Fig. 8.1).

E. H. Wilkes (✉) · G. M. Woodward
Department of Clinical Biochemistry, University College London Hospitals, London, UK
e-mail: edmund.wilkes@nhs.net

G. Rumsby, G. M. Woodward (eds.), *Disorders of Steroidogenesis*,
https://doi.org/10.1007/978-3-319-96364-8_8

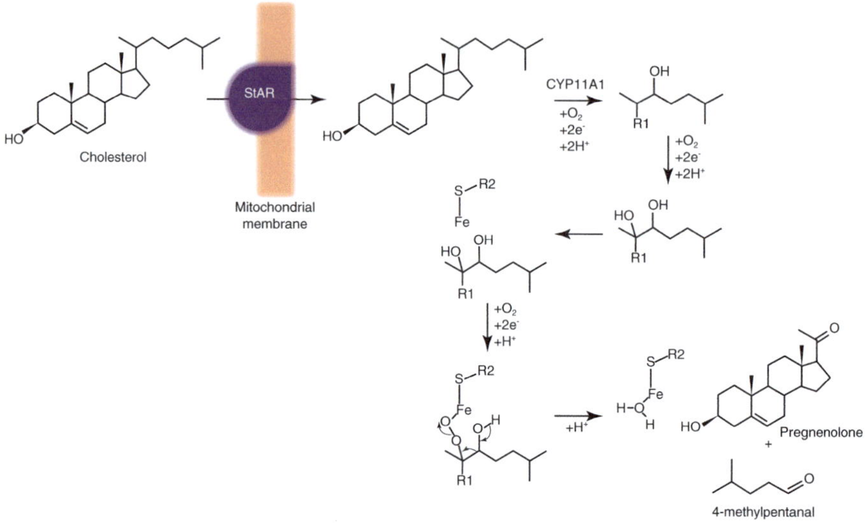

Fig. 8.1 Cholesterol is transported across the mitochondrial membrane in a process facilitated by StAR, where it interacts with CYP11A1, adrenodoxin and adrenodoxin reductase. The reaction products are pregnenolone and 4-methylpentanal. R1 represents the steroid nucleus and R2 represents the Cys423 residue within CYP11A1. The Fe atom is coordinated within the haem group associated with CYP11A1

The uptake of cholesterol into the mitochondria is stimulated by trophic hormones – ACTH in the adrenal and LH in the gonads – by a cAMP-mediated mechanism and requires synthesis of new StAR protein. The protein is also upregulated by phosphorylation on amino acid Ser195 by protein kinase A.

CYP11A1, also commonly referred to as cholesterol 20-22 lyase, is the rate-limiting step of steroidogenesis. Indeed, the amount of steroid present within a cell is dependent on the regulation and expression of CYP11A1 by ACTH and angiotensin II in the adrenal gland and by LH in the gonads. CYP11A1 interacts with adrenodoxin and adrenodoxin reductase to form the cholesterol side-chain cleavage complex. Cholesterol side-chain cleavage occurs as a series of reactions that result in the hydroxylation of carbons 20α and 20 (requiring four electrons transferred from adrenodoxin and adrenodoxin reductase from NAPDH molecules) and the breakage of the C20–C22 carbon–carbon bond (Fig. 8.1).

The CYP11A1 enzyme is present in all steroidogenic tissues, including the placenta. It is not clear what mechanism is used to promote cholesterol uptake in the placenta, as StAR is not present in this tissue.

Lipoid congenital adrenal hyperplasia (LCAH) is a rare, severe form of congenital adrenal hyperplasia (CAH) and, as with the other forms of CAH, is an autosomal recessive disorder. It is caused by mutations in the StAR protein. A small amount of cholesterol is still transported into the mitochondria through StAR-independent mechanisms, and thus a low level of steroidogenesis is maintained; however, this is at levels insufficient to maintain normal physiology and leads to compensatory activation of pro-steroidogenic stimuli (e.g. renin and ACTH secretion). LCAH develops in two stages; the so-called 'two-hit' hypothesis. Firstly, there is an increase in the amount of low-density lipoprotein cholesterol being trafficked into adrenal cells and increased *de novo* cholesterol production resulting in an accumulation of lipid in the cytoplasm. Secondly, the accumulated cholesterol esters cause oxidative damage and cell death, with complete abrogation of steroidogenesis.

Deficiency of CYP11A1 was initially thought to be incompatible with life, as the enzyme is required for placental progesterone synthesis from the second trimester of pregnancy after the maternal corpus luteum regresses. There are, however, cases now described that have survived to term. In contrast to StAR deficiency, lipid accumulation does not usually occur, and the adrenals are not hyperplastic, but tend to be rather hypoplastic.

8.2 Presentation

The clinical presentation of LCAH is entirely as a consequence of the affected individual's inability to produce mineralocorticoids, glucocorticoids and sex steroids and usually occurs in the first few weeks of life. The most common presentation is with symptoms of adrenal failure. Low levels of circulating mineralocorticoids lead to severe hyponatraemia, hyperkalaemia and, potentially, metabolic acidosis. Inadequate levels of circulating glucocorticoids also contribute to hyponatraemia and hyperkalaemia, in addition to causing hypoglycaemia and a failure to thrive. Hyperpigmentation is also a common finding in affected individuals due to the compensatory upregulation of ACTH (and therefore α-melanocyte-stimulating hormone) secretion in an attempt to drive the adrenals to produce cortisol. Partial loss of StAR activity may present later in life and in some cases can be mistaken for familial glucocorticoid insufficiency, as mineralocorticoid production is preserved.

The clinical impact of the lack of sex steroids differs depending on whether the affected individual is a karyotypic male (XY) or female (XX). Due to failure of the Leydig cells of the fetal testis to produce adequate androgens in utero, male patients often present with female genitalia at birth – i.e. it is a 46XY disorder of sex development (DSD). Testicular damage is present at birth. In contrast, because the ovaries are not stimulated to produce significant oestrogens until puberty, they are initially spared. Cholesterol accumulation does however occur in the recruited and stimulated follicle, eventually leading to its failure in the later phases of ovarian steroid production. Unstimulated follicles remain undamaged. Thus, due to the oestrogens produced during early follicular development, female LCAH patients can have normal breast development and menses. Due to progressive damage to the recruited follicles in each cycle, however, progesterone is not produced in any significant quantity, and the cycles remain anovulatory. Despite the differences in the disease manifestation at birth, both male and female patients fail to produce dehydroepiandrosterone (DHEA) in utero, and thus maternal circulating levels of oestriol are reduced. The amount of circulating progesterone, normally produced by the fetal cells of the placenta, is also reduced – the effects of which being largely undetermined.

CYP11A1 deficiency also typically presents as adrenal failure but has a variable phenotype ranging from a 46XY DSD to isolated adrenal insufficiency. The most common presenting feature is hypoglycaemia and adrenal failure; however, the majority of cases have presented outside of the neonatal period. The adrenal glands tend to be normal or small in size in contrast to LCAH. Genital development can be very variable ranging from female to hypospadias with hypogonadism in 46XY patients.

8.3 Genetics

The *STARD1* gene which endodes for the StAR protein is composed of seven exons and is located on chromosome 8p11.2. At least 40 mutations have been identified, a considerable number of which occur in the C-terminal (exons 5–7) which encodes the sterol-binding domain. Two variants, p.Arg182Leu and p.Gln258Ter, are relatively common; the first found in 78% of affected alleles from Palestinian patients and the second in 80% of affected alleles from Japanese and Korean patients. Later presenting cases of the disease tend to have mutations that retain 10–25% of StAR activity. These milder forms have less severe hyponatraemia, milder elevations in renin and detectable aldosterone levels, and are sometimes referred to as 'non-classical' LCAH.

CYP11A1, encoding the cholesterol side-chain cleavage enzyme, has been mapped to chromosome 15q23-q24 and has nine exons. Some of the pathological variants encode proteins with essentially no activity, and it has been hypothesised that the only way the child could have survived in utero is by extended maintenance of the corpus luteum in pregnancy beyond the second trimester. One mutation, p.Arg451Trp, was found in an adrenal-only phenotype with normal androgen production. In vitro studies demonstrated that the enzyme had a catalytic efficiency of approximately 20% of the wild-type enzyme. This degree of enzyme activity was presumably adequate for testosterone synthesis in utero although, postnatally, testicular response to human chorionic gonadotrophin stimulation was inadequate.

Genetic diagnosis is essential for accurate confirmation of these disorders and to permit family studies.

8.4 Diagnosis

For patients presenting with symptoms of adrenal failure in childhood, CAH is an important differential diagnosis. Various endocrinological investigations are useful in the diagnosis of LCAH and CYP11A1 deficiency, which invariably all demonstrate low levels of adrenal steroids. Alongside these single tests, dynamic function tests such as the short Synacthen and human chorionic gonadotrophin (hCG) stimulation tests can be used to assess adrenal reserve and gonadal function, respectively. In those with LCAH and CYP11A1 deficiency, adrenal cortisol production will show little or no response to Synacthen. If salt losing, renin and aldosterone should be assessed. Male patients with LCAH will also show little or no testosterone response to hCG stimulation.

A urine steroid profile can be carried out to exclude other forms of CAH and will show minimal steroid production and no abnormal intermediates.

Adrenal ultrasound will show enlarged adrenals in LCAH but normal or small glands in CYP11A1 deficiency. A karyotype should be performed to determine the genetic sex.

8.5 Case Study

A 15-year-old female presented with primary amenorrhoea. Past clinical history included an episode of salt wasting at 2 years of age, with documented hyponatraemia and hyperkalaemia that were treated with fludrocortisone and hydrocortisone. On examination as a teenager, she was found to have an absent uterus. The karyotype was 46XY. A urine steroid profile was sent for analysis while on treatment.

The profile was notable for an absence of adrenal androgens. There were no abnormal metabolites to indicate 17α-hydroxylase or 3β-hydroxysteroid dehydrogenase deficiencies as an underlying cause of androgen failure, although metabolites may have been suppressed by concurrent hydrocortisone treatment. An early disorder of steroidogenesis could not be excluded biochemically; however, genetic testing subsequently confirmed StAR deficiency, finding homozygosity for a mutation in the *STARD1* gene.

8.6 Steroid Profile

A urine steroid profile is a useful tool; it can be used to include or exclude all forms of CAH and other disorders of steroidogenesis simultaneously. As all steroid synthesis is impaired in both LCAH and CYP11A1 deficiency, a urine steroid profile will show a potentially normal pattern but low levels of all their respective metabolites. A word of caution, however: if a random sample is from a neonate, the sample may be very dilute or of insufficient volume to give an adequate response. Assessment of urine creatinine can therefore aid interpretation. In contrast to other forms of CAH, there are no specific metabolites that can discriminate between LCAH and CYP11A deficiency. In the late presenting case described above (Sec. 8.5), treatment could not be withheld; however, the adrenal androgens were markedly reduced and therefore provided a clue to the diagnosis (Fig. 8.2).

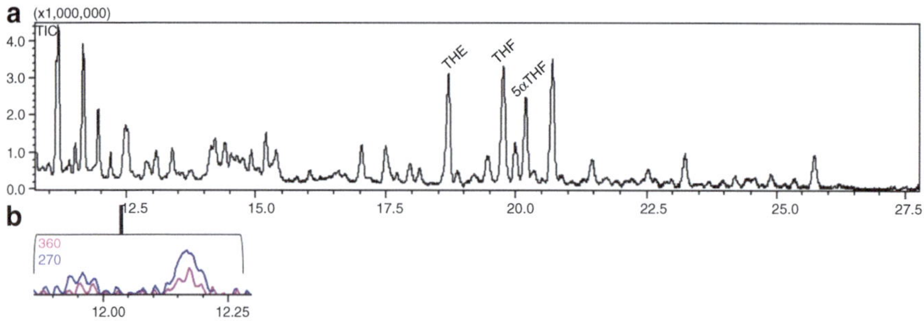

Fig. 8.2 (**a**) Urine steroid profile from a 15-year-old patient with StAR deficiency. Cortisol metabolites are present as patient is on treatment, but there are minimal adrenal androgen metabolites, androsterone and aetiocholanolone, that can only be picked up by selective ion scan with ions at m/z 360 and 270 as shown in (**b**)

8.7 Treatment

The adrenal insufficiency resulting from defects in early steroidogenesis is treated through the pharmacological replacement of glucocorticoids and mineralocorticoids. The Endocrine Society guidelines recommend hydrocortisone or cortisone acetate in three divided doses per day. Prednisolone, administered once or twice a day, can be used as an alternative, but dexamethasone is not recommended due to difficulties titrating the dose and the risk of side effects of glucocorticoid excess. The dose does not need to be as high as for virilising forms of CAH because there is no excess androgen production. Fludrocortisone is required for mineralocorticoid replacement and can be monitored by measurement of plasma renin. Treatment should be monitored clinically through the assessment of clinical parameters such as weight and blood pressure.

Further Reading

StAR-Related Domain

Tsuijhita Y, Hurley JH. Structure and lipid transport mechanism of a StAR-related domain. Nat Struct Biol. 2000;7:408–14.

Steroid Synthesis from Cholesterol

Miller WL. Role of mitochondria in steroidogenesis. Endocr Dev. 2011;20:1–19.

Strushkevich N, MacKenzie F, Cherkesova T, Grabovec I, Usanov S, Park H-W. Structural basis for pregnenolone biosynthesis by the mitochondrial monooxygenase system. Proc Natl Acad Sci U S A. 2011;108(25):10139–43.

Genetics

Tee MK, Abramsohn M, Loewenthal N, et al. Varied clinical presentation of seven patients with mutations in the CYP11A1 encoding the cholesterol side-chain cleavage enzyme, P450scc. J Clin Endocrinol Metab. 2013;98:713–20.

Pathophysiology

King SR, Bhangoo A, Stocco DM. Functional and physiological consequences of StAR deficiency: role in lipoid congenital adrenal hyperplasia. Endocr Dev. 2011;20:47–53.

Hauffa B, Hiort O. P450 side-chain cleavage deficiency—a rare cause of congenital adrenal hyperplasia. Endocr Dev. 2010;20:54–62.

Aldosterone Synthase Deficiency

9

Oliver Clifford-Mobley

9.1 Introduction

Aldosterone synthase (cytochrome P450, subfamily 11B, polypeptide 2) is a mitochondrial enzyme that catalyses the last three steps in the biosynthesis of aldosterone: 11β-hydroxylation, 18β-hydroxylation and 18-oxidation (Fig. 9.1). This enzyme is localised to the zona glomerulosa of the adrenal cortex, and aldosterone production occurs only in this outer layer of the adrenal gland. The gene which encodes aldosterone synthase is *CYP11B2*. This gene has a very similar coding sequence to *CYP11B1*, the gene for steroid 11β-hydroxylase, which catalyses the last step in the biosynthesis of cortisol (the two enzymes have 93% protein sequence homology). Although the two genes are similar, they have different 5′ sequences, which allows for their separate regulation by angiotensin II and ACTH, respectively, and their expression is localised to separate parts of the adrenal cortex. Aldosterone is termed a mineralocorticoid because of its function of maintaining salt and fluid balance. It is important to recognise that, although aldosterone is the most potent mineralocorticoid, other adrenal steroids also have some mineralocorticoid activity; the most important of these are 11-deoxycorticosterone and cortisol.

Aldosterone synthase deficiency is unique compared to the other inborn errors of adrenal steroid biosynthesis in that its phenotype involves only disturbances in salt and fluid handling and not in either cortisol synthesis or sexual differentiation (as occurs in congenital adrenal hyperplasia, CAH). Aldosterone production is independent from the hypothalamic-pituitary-adrenal axis, and patients with aldosterone synthase deficiency can produce cortisol normally; therefore no increased

O. Clifford-Mobley
Department of Clinical Biochemistry, University Hospitals Bristol NHS Foundation Trust, Bristol, UK
e-mail: oliver.clifford-mobley@nhs.net

G. Rumsby, G. M. Woodward (eds.), *Disorders of Steroidogenesis*,
https://doi.org/10.1007/978-3-319-96364-8_9

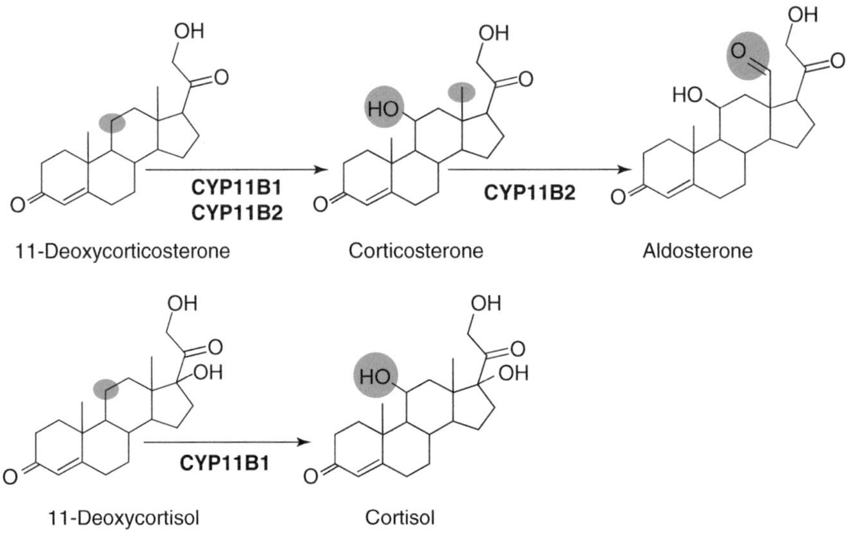

Fig. 9.1 Enzymatic reaction catalysed by 11β-hydroxylase (CYP11B1) and aldosterone synthase (CYP11B2)

ACTH drive to the adrenal occurs, and there is no increased flux down the sex steroid biosynthetic pathways. Aldosterone instead is regulated via the renin-angiotensin-aldosterone system (RAAS, Fig. 9.2). In the absence of aldosterone, the kidneys are unable to adequately retain sodium or excrete potassium. Consequently excess sodium and water is lost in the urine and hypovolaemia occurs. In the presence of hypovolaemia, normal physiological osmoregulation is overridden, and there is an increase in antidiuretic hormone (ADH) secretion. This leads to retention of free water at the expense of a reduced osmolality. The key biochemical features of untreated aldosterone synthase deficiency are hyponatraemia and hyperkalaemia.

Because aldosterone synthase has both 18β-hydroxylase and 18-oxidase activities, deficiency of this enzyme is sometimes subdivided into defects in either catalytic activity: these are termed corticosterone methyl oxidase (CMO) type 1 and type 2, respectively. Whilst this distinction is of interest to the biochemist in light of the different steroid metabolites seen, it does not alter the phenotype and is of little clinical relevance.

9.2 Presentation

Aldosterone synthase deficiency should be considered in an infant with unexplained hypovolaemia, hyponatraemia or hyperkalaemia. The severity of symptoms generally varies as a function of age, and adults are much better able to tolerate it. Infants are unable to replace the lost salt on their own; in contrast the ready availability of

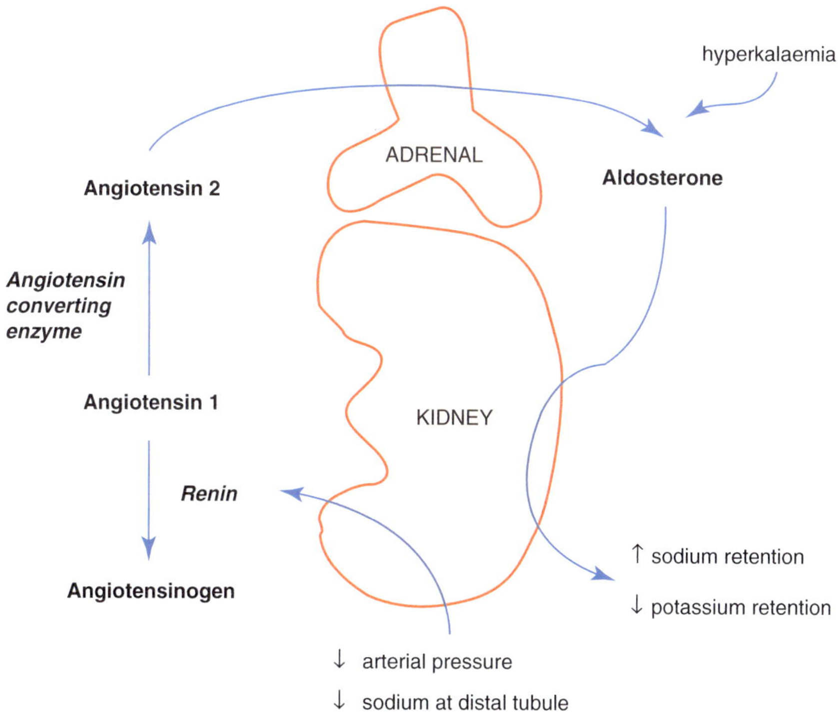

Fig. 9.2 The renin-angiotensin-aldosterone system. A reduction in the flow of filtrate, or in its sodium concentration, at the juxtaglomerular apparatus is the stimulus for renin secretion. This peptidase converts angiotensinogen to angiotensin 1 in the circulation, which is in turn converted to angiotensin 2 by angiotensin converting enzyme. Angiotensin 2 and also hyperkalaemia stimulate the production of aldosterone in the zona glomerulosa of the adrenal cortex. Aldosterone travels to the kidney where it binds to the mineralocorticoid receptor in the distal tubule and promotes the reabsorption of sodium and with it the concomitant transfer of water and the excretion of potassium

salt in a normal diet makes this easier for an adult, and the presence of a salt appetite in affected patients helps. The mineralocorticoid effect of other adrenal steroids also plays a role in mitigating the clinical presentation of aldosterone synthase deficiency. Therefore, adults with aldosterone synthase deficiency may be asymptomatic, although isolated hyperkalaemia and symptomatic salt-loss in adulthood have been reported.

9.3 Genetics

CYP11B2 and *CYP11B1* are located approximately 40 kilobases apart on chromosome 8q24.3 and share more than 95% similarity in nucleotide coding sequence. Construction of *CYP11B1-CYP11B2* hybrids has shown that the sequences important for the final 18-oxidation step unique to aldosterone synthase are encoded by amino acids at 288, 296, 302, 325 and 320 located in exons 5 and 6.

Loss of function variants in *CYP11B2* are known to cause aldosterone synthase deficiency. Due to the rarity of the disease, there are no overall common mutations, though within specific ethnic groups there may be common mutations due to founder effects. The missense variants p.Val386Ala and p.Arg173Lys are polymorphic in many populations. However, when p.Val386Ala occurs in combination with other missense changes, notably p.Arg181Trp (as occurs in the Iranian-Jewish population) and p.Glu198Asp, there is a deleterious effect on protein function leading to symptomatic aldosterone synthase deficiency. This finding suggests a more complex relationship between protein structure and catalytic activity. Furthermore, there is not a clear genotype-biochemical phenotype correlation for CMO1 and CMO2. For example, the Iranian-Jewish population with p.Val386Ala and p.Arg181Trp have CMO2, characterised by elevated levels of 18-hydroxycorticosterone, and in vitro enzyme studies show the expected selectively reduced 18-oxidation activity of this double mutant. The p.Val386Ala and p.Glu198Asp double mutant behaves similarly in vitro, but patients with this genotype have been described as CMO1.

The observation of patients with clinical and biochemical features of aldosterone synthase deficiency, but without any pathological variants in *CYP11B2*, has posed the question whether any further genes may be implicated in the pathogenesis of this disease. This is as yet unknown.

Errors in recombination can lead to a *CYP11B1-B2* hybrid construct in which aldosterone synthesis occurs in the zona fasciculata under ACTH regulation. This chimaera underlies the disorder of glucocorticoid remedial hyperaldosteronism (GRA) and is discussed in more detail in Chap. 5.

9.4 Diagnosis

Urine steroid profile is not the most sensitive technique for measuring aldosterone metabolites (see section on urine steroid profile below). Measurement of both aldosterone and renin in blood is an essential investigation to assess the integrity of the RAAS axis. Renin is commonly measured either as its enzymatic activity or as its protein mass. Traditionally the former approach is viewed as superior because it is the catalytic activity of renin that affects regulation of RAAS, and also a lower limit of quantitation is possible than with current renin mass assays. In the setting of suspected aldosterone synthase deficiency, an elevated renin is to be expected, and using a mass assay is acceptable. Results supportive of aldosterone synthase deficiency are hyperreninaemic hypoaldosteronism in the presence of a salt-losing state. Normal levels of aldosterone and renin are much higher in the first 6 months of life, possibly relating to tubular immaturity. Therefore, results must be interpreted using age-specific reference ranges if available or at least with this knowledge in mind.

The normal physiological response to a salt-losing state is hyperreninaemic hyperaldosteronism, and if this is the case, then alternative diagnoses should be considered including the inherited tubulopathies (e.g. Bartter syndrome, Dent disease), pseudohypoaldosteronism and defects in the mineralocorticoid receptor.

If hyperreninaemic hypoaldosteronism is confirmed, this supports aldosterone synthase deficiency, but other causes of primary adrenal insufficiency should be excluded. This can be done by assessing cortisol reserve with a short synacthen test: a normal response is expected in aldosterone synthase deficiency. The enzymes which are defective in two forms of CAH, 21-hydroxylase and 3β-hydroxysteroid dehydrogenase, are required for aldosterone synthesis, so these inborn errors can also cause salt-loss. Both can be excluded by urine steroid profile analysis. Addison's disease also presents with a salt-losing crisis. Steroid 11-hydroxylase deficiency, whilst normally considered a hypertensive form of CAH, can present with a salt-losing crisis in infancy. This disorder can also be excluded by urine steroid profile.

Other commonly measured steroid hormones and intermediates (e.g., cortisol, androstenedione, 17-hydroxyprogesterone) should be normal in aldosterone synthase deficiency because the defective enzyme is specific to the mineralocorticoid pathway and is not involved in the biosynthesis of any other steroids. Measurement of the specific precursors of aldosterone in blood can be performed, though these are not commonly available investigations. Elevated 11-deoxycorticosterone indicates an increased flux down the aldosterone biosynthetic pathway and will be present in aldosterone synthase deficiency but may also be found in salt-losing states due to other conditions. By measuring 18-hydroxycorticosterone and aldosterone, a biochemical distinction between CMO1 and CMO2 can be made. In CMO1 both steroids will be very low, if present at all, whereas in CMO2 the ratio of 18-hydroxycorticosterone to aldosterone will be grossly elevated.

During a salt-losing episode serum biochemistry may demonstrate hyponatraemia as the kidneys retain free water under the influence of ADH in an effort to maintain circulating volume. Hyperkalaemia and acidosis are common findings because the normal action of aldosterone is to retain sodium at the expense of potassium and hydrogen ions. Urine analysis will show inappropriately high urine sodium.

9.5 Case Study

An infant was born at term to unrelated parents. Birth weight was on the 25th centile, but this continued to fall, and at 3 months the child was investigated for failure to thrive. Serum sodium was 126 mmol/L and potassium 6.2 mmol/L with urine sodium 34 mmol/L. Serum cortisol was 1152 nmol/L following Synacthen stimulation excluding a salt-losing form of CAH. Aldosterone was 1160 pmol/L (reference range up to 2000) and renin activity 19 pmol/mL/h (reference range <10), thus aldosterone was inappropriately low suggestive of impaired synthesis.

Urine steroid profile showed an increase of corticosterone metabolites, whilst tetrahydroaldosterone was undetectable. High levels of 18-hydroxylated corticosterone metabolites were seen consistent with CMO2. Genetic testing found homozygosity for p.Arg181Pro missense change predicted to be pathogenic. The parents were heterozygous for the same variant.

9.6 Steroid Profile

Aldosterone exists in two circulating forms due to the nonenzymatic formation of an hemiacetal. Both forms are metabolised by 5α-reductase and 3α-hydroxysteroid dehydrogenase to tetrahydro derivatives, and these are the major urinary metabolites (Fig. 9.3). However, these are not normally visible in a urine steroid profile because there is a much lower production of aldosterone required to maintain euvolaemia than is required of the other adrenal steroids for their own physiological functions. Normal serum aldosterone concentration is in the hundreds of picomolar range, whereas, for example, a normal cortisol is in the hundreds of nanomolar range, a difference of three orders of magnitude.

The immediate precursor of aldosterone is corticosterone (known as compound B); its major urinary metabolite αTHB is formed by the action of 5α-reductase and 3α-hydroxysteroid dehydrogenase. In normal salt-replete states, this is the only

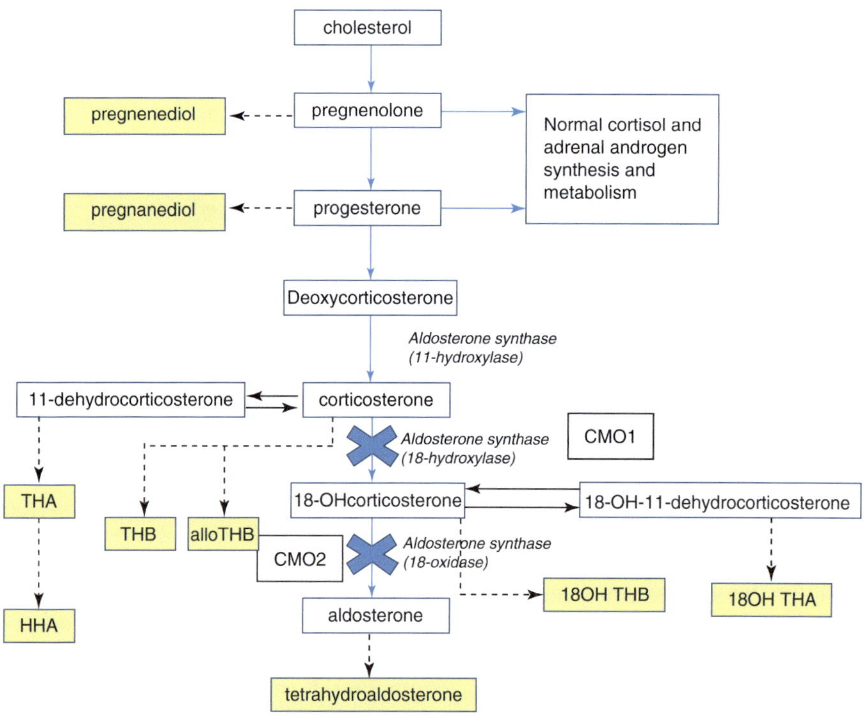

Fig. 9.3 Origin of urine metabolites seen in aldosterone synthase deficiency and pseudohypoaldosteronism. Cortisol and adrenal androgen production are unaffected. Corticosterone and, in CMO2, 18-hydroxycorticosterone metabolites are produced in excess, presumably as a result of the action of CYP11B1 on deoxycorticosterone and corticosterone, respectively. CMO1 is characterised by low 18-hydroxycorticosterone whereas in CMO2 this metabolite is elevated. In pseudohypoaldosteronism, aldosterone is produced in excess and aldosterone metabolites may also be detected

Table 9.1 Steroid metabolites seen in aldosterone synthase deficiency, retention times (methylene units, MU) of their MO-TMS derivatives and characteristic ions (see appendix for spectra)

Steroid	Trivial name	MU	Relevant ions
5β-Pregnan-3α,21-diol-11,20-dione	Tetrahydro-11-dehydrocorticosterone (THA)	29.77	400, 188
5β-Pregnan-3α,11β,21-triol-20-one	Tetrahydrocorticosterone (THB)	30.00/30.16	564, 188
11β,18-epoxy-3α,18,21-trihydroxy-5β-pregnan-20-one	Tetrahydroaldosterone hemiacetal	29.50/29.76	506, 416
5α-Pregnan-3α,11β,21-triol-20-one	Allo-tetrahydrocorticosterone (alloTHB)	30.16/30.80	474, 188
5β-Pregnan-3α,18, 21-triol-11,20-dione	18-OHTHA	30.64/31.44	578, 457
3α,11β,21-trihydroxy-5β-pregnan-20-on-18-al	Tetrahydroaldosterone	30.86/30.91	607, 535
5β-Pregnan-3α,6α,21-triol-11,20-dione	6αOH-tetrahydroTHA	31.52	519, 188

metabolite from the aldosterone biosynthetic pathway that is found in a urine steroid profile (for the same reason as described above). The observation of any mineralocorticoid metabolite other than αTHB should be followed up by more careful interrogation of the steroid profile (Table 9.1).

The equivalent 5β-reduced form of corticosterone is also sometimes seen. Corticosterone is reduced to 11-dehydrocorticosterone (known as compound A) by 11β-hydroxysteroid dehydrogenase type 2. Metabolism of 11-dehydrocorticosterone to αTHA and βTHA occurs analogously to the metabolism of corticosterone. Further metabolites include 6- and 18-hydroxylated THA and THB and hexahydro metabolites formed by the action of 20α- or 20β-hydroxysteroid dehydrogenase. It is in the pattern of urine steroid metabolites that the distinction between CMO1 and CMO2 can be seen. The fundamental difference is the presence of elevated levels of 18-hydroxylated metabolites in CMO2, but not in CMO1 (see Fig. 9.4). A common ion with $m/z = 188$, derived from 21-hydroxy, 20-oxo, 17-deoxy with no additional functional groups on the steroid D ring, is found in the electron impact mass spectra of several metabolites of corticosterone (see Table 9.1). Therefore, inspection of an extracted ion spectrum at this m/z is a useful method for picking up the low levels of these steroids and is to be recommended in all urine steroid profiles with clinical details of unexplained salt-loss.

Symptomatic salt-loss due to any cause will increase the drive to produce aldosterone and will be evident from increased excretion of corticosterone metabolites (Fig. 9.5). In aldosterone synthase deficiency due to CMO1, there will not be any excretion of aldosterone metabolites, although aldosterone is sometimes found in CMO2. However, due to the inherent insensitivity of urine steroid profile and the low concentration of aldosterone, it may be hard to distinguish aldosterone synthase deficiency from another cause of salt-loss, and therefore blood renin and aldosterone measurement is required (see section on diagnosis above).

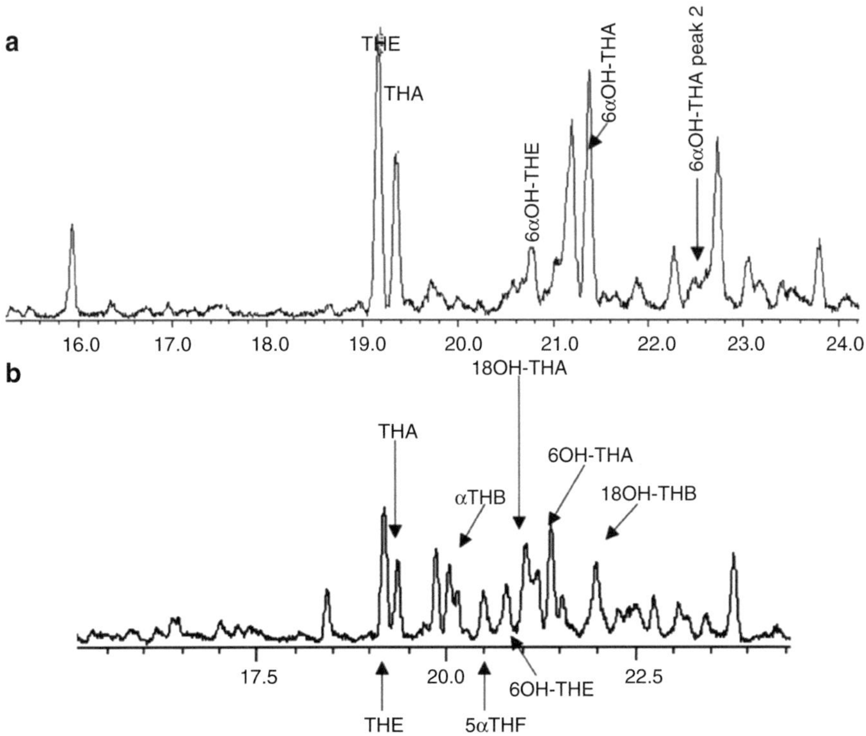

Fig. 9.4 Examples of urine steroid profiles from two patients with aldosterone synthase deficiency showing (**a**) complete loss of CYP11B2 enzyme activity (CMO1) and (**b**) loss of 18-hydroxysteroid dehydrogenase activity (CMO2). In both cases normal cortisol metabolites are present. CMO2 is characterised by the presence of 18-hydroxylated metabolites. Neonatal metabolites of cortisol (6OHTHE) and corticosterone (6OH-THA) are both present

In a patient with aldosterone synthase deficiency, replacement of salt and fluid has the effect of switching off the renin drive. The production of the aldosterone precursors drops rapidly, and therefore a characteristic pattern of urine steroid excretion may not be found. This caveat applies to all inborn errors of adrenal steroid biosynthesis; however, in the case of aldosterone synthase deficiency, the effect is particularly marked due to the low physiological concentrations of aldosterone precursors. Therefore, the diagnostic urine sample must be collected during a salt-losing crisis. From a laboratory perspective, it is imperative that if the clinical details state salt-loss, then the profile should be closely inspected for corticosterone metabolites which may only be present in trace amounts.

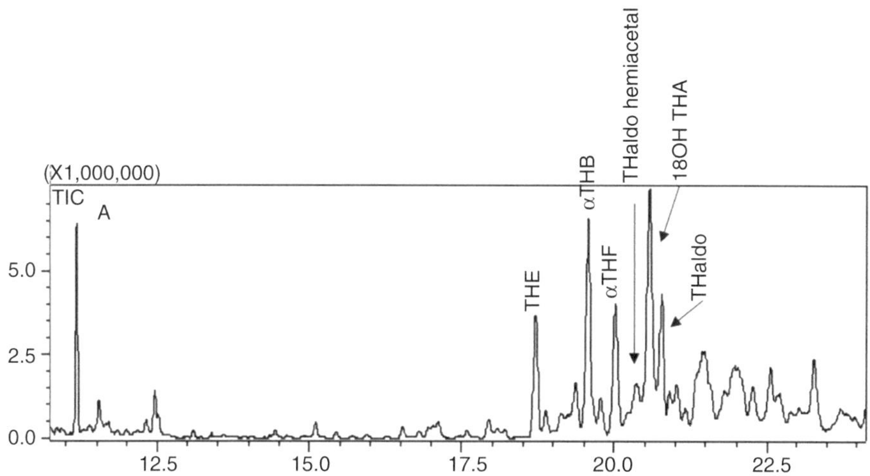

Fig. 9.5 Urine steroid profile from a case of pseudohypoaldosteronism. In contrast to aldosterone synthase deficiency, aldosterone metabolites are present when the sample is taken during a salt-losing crisis, along with elevated corticosterone metabolites. In the case of urinary tract infections, cholesterol may also be present

9.7 Treatment

CYP11B2 deficiency requires mineralocorticoid replacement therapy usually with fludrocortisone, and monitoring can be done by measurement of plasma renin. Cortisol biosynthesis is not affected and does not require replacement.

Further Reading

Bassett MH, White PC, Rainey WE. The regulation of aldosterone synthase expression. Mol Cell Endocrinol. 2004;217:67–74.

White PC. Aldosterone synthase deficiency and related disorders. Mol Cell Endocrinol. 2004;217:81–7.

17β-Hydroxysteroid Dehydrogenase Deficiency

10

Gill Rumsby

10.1 Introduction

There are now 12 known members of the 17β-hydroxysteroid dehydrogenase (17βHSD) family of enzymes, not all of which have been found in humans. Some play a role in the formation of the active steroids, e.g. oestradiol and testosterone, by catalysing the conversion of an inactive keto residue to an active hydroxyl; others are involved in steroid inactivation usually by the reverse, dehydrogenation reaction. Most of these enzymes are members of the short-chain dehydrogenase/reductase family of proteins, but at least one, 17βHSD type 5 (also known as AKR1C3), is a member of the aldo-keto reductase family. The short-chain reductases are multimeric enzymes that share several amino acid sequence motifs, particularly those that are involved with cofactor binding, but otherwise have a very low sequence homology. These enzymes are encoded by different genes and may be expressed in different tissues as well as have different substrate and cofactor preferences.

While reactions have been shown to be reversible in vitro, this is unlikely to be the case in vivo where the concentration of cofactors is limited. It is now appreciated that those 17βHSD that play a reductive role, i.e. converting the ketone to hydroxyl group, have a preference for NADPH as cofactor, while enzymes with an oxidative role prefer NAD^+. This preference presumably reflects the intracellular levels of these cofactors: the cytosolic ratio of NAD^+/NADH is approximately 1000:1, whereas $NADP^+$/NADPH is 1:100. The odd-numbered 17βHSD enzymes, types 1, 3, 5 and 7, catalyse the reduction reaction, while types 2, 4 and 8 catalyse oxidation of substrates. The role of the different types of 17βHSD enzymes in human steroid hormone biosynthesis is shown in Fig. 10.1.

G. Rumsby
Department of Clinical Biochemistry, University College London Hospitals, London, UK
e-mail: gill.rumsby@nhs.net

G. Rumsby, G. M. Woodward (eds.), *Disorders of Steroidogenesis*,
https://doi.org/10.1007/978-3-319-96364-8_10

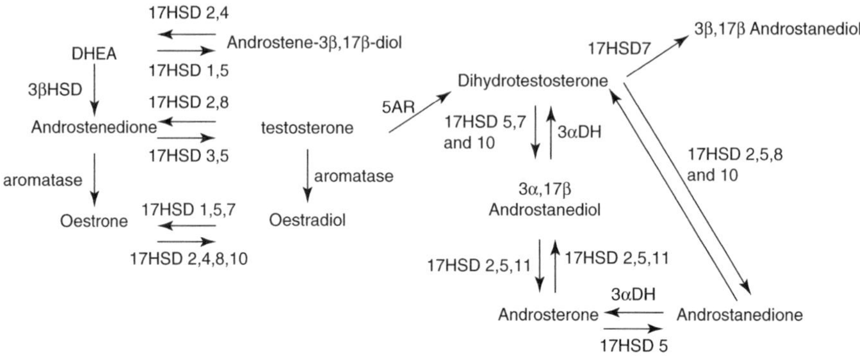

Fig. 10.1 The role of different 17βHSD enzymes in human steroid hormone metabolism. 5AR, 5α reductase; 3αDH, 3α hydroxysteroid dehydrogenase

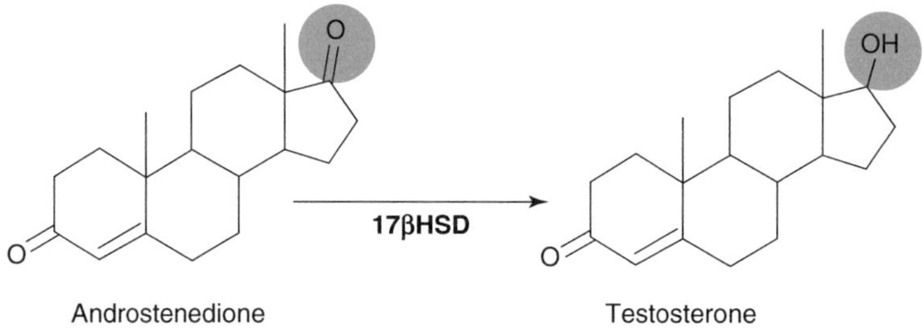

Fig. 10.2 The activation of androstenedione to testosterone by reduction of the oxo group at carbon 17 of the steroid molecule catalysed by 17βHSD3

17βHSD enzymes are expressed in a wide variety of tissues including the placenta, ovary and testis as well as adipose tissue, liver, lung, skin, breast and red blood cells. The important enzyme from the point of view of disorders of sex development (DSD) is the type 3 enzyme, expressed at highest levels in the testis. This enzyme catalyses the conversion of androstenedione to the active steroid testosterone by reduction of the keto group at carbon 17 of the steroid molecule (Fig. 10.2).

Enzyme deficiency leads to impaired testosterone synthesis in utero and consequently poor or absent virilisation of a 46XY male. In the fetus the development of the Wolffian ducts from the bipotential gonad is triggered by expression of a number of genes including *WT1* and *NR5A1* encoding steroidogenic factor (SF1). SF1 plays a number of roles including the transcriptional regulation of steroid-synthesising enzymes and regulation of anti-Müllerian hormone production by the primordial Sertoli cells. In the XY gonad, expression of *SRY* (sex-determining region on the Y) leads to the increased expression of the SOX9 transcription factor in the Sertoli cells in synergy with SF1 and differentiation of the male genital tract with development of the male internal genitalia, i.e. epididymis, vas deferens and seminal vesicles.

Testosterone is also thought to play a role in Wolffian duct development. Somewhat surprisingly then, this process still occurs in individuals with 17βHSD3 deficiency who are theoretically unable to produce testicular testosterone and also in those with androgen insensitivity who have defects in the androgen receptor and therefore cannot respond to testosterone. Consequently, the presence of well-differentiated Wolffian duct structures cannot be used to differentiate between these two disorders. The possibility is therefore raised that either the fetal androgen receptor can respond to the increased androstenedione produced or there is some other means of synthesising fetal testosterone from the elevated intra-testicular androstenedione concentrations. Studies using a transactivation assay have shown that androstenedione at concentrations >10 nM, a concentration likely to be exceeded in the testis of affected patients, can activate the androgen receptor at least in vitro. The role of other 17βHSD enzymes in either the testis or extra-testicular tissues is also postulated. From animal studies there is evidence the mouse fetal (but not adult) Leydig cell lacks 17βHSD3, and therefore its primary product is androstenedione that is metabolised to testosterone in murine Sertoli cells that express both 17βHSD1 and 3; thus the two cell types appear to cooperate to synthesise testosterone. There is however no evidence for 17βHSD1 playing such a role in human testicular testosterone synthesis as the enzyme is said to be more selective, catalysing the conversion oestrone to oestradiol only.

10.2 Presentation

Deficiency of 17βHSD3 is a rare form of DSD but in our adult 46XY DSD cohort accounts for approximately 25% cases—a similar number to those caused by 5α-reductase deficiency. The incidence of the disease in the Netherlands was calculated to be in the order of 1:143,000 newborns, i.e. less frequent than that of androgen insensitivity syndrome (1:99,000), and with a carrier frequency of 1 in 135. In areas of high consanguinity, the incidence can be as high as 1 in 200–300. Combining data from published series, the majority of genetic males, i.e. 46XY, with this disorder appear female at birth with inguinal masses occurring in approximately one-third. These individuals have female external genitalia with a blind-ending vagina and separate opening for the vagina and urethra, and the sex of rearing will be female. The Müllerian ducts are absent consistent with normal fetal testicular Sertoli cell production of anti-Müllerian hormone. Thus, the prepubertal phenotype is similar to that of androgen insensitivity syndrome that results from defects in the androgen receptor, and the disorder may only come to notice when the female fails to go into puberty.

Virilisation occurs in approximately 30% of cases with intact testes at puberty. Changes include rugged, pigmented skin of the labia majora, clitoromegaly, male pattern baldness and voice lowering. The virilisation is believed to be due to conversion of the excess androstenedione to testosterone by other 17βHSD enzymes, most likely 17βHSD5 that is expressed in the Leydig cells. Thus, the phenotype overlaps with that of 5α-reductase deficiency. It is therefore highly likely that incorrect diagnoses may occur if appropriate biochemical and genetic testing is not performed.

Females, i.e. 46XX genotype, with genetically confirmed 17βHSD3 deficiency are asymptomatic and endocrinologically normal. There have been some reports of infertility, but as the enzyme is not expressed in ovarian tissue, this may be a completely unrelated finding.

10.3 Genetics

The gene encoding 17βHSD3, *HSD17B3*, is located on the long arm of chromosome 9 at 9q22. It contains 11 exons spread over 78 kb, encoding a protein of 310 amino acids. A number of mutations have been described to date including missense, minor deletions and some recurring splice site mutations that lead to exon skipping. It should be noted that the DNA nomenclature used in this chapter is that recommended by the Human Genome Variation Society (www.hgvs.org/) and may differ from that in the original publications. The c.277+4A>T and c.607-1G>A splice site mutations and the two missense changes, p.Asp74Thr and p.Arg80Gln, are found worldwide and possibly reflect founder mutations. In the case of c.277+4A>T, a common haplotype was found suggesting that the mutation originated in Europe and was subsequently spread to the United States and Australia by migration. The c.607-1G>A is found in those of Turkish, Greek and Syrian ancestry. De novo mutations have also been described. Some of the missense mutations have been expressed in vitro and confirm that there is minimal activity of the mutant protein. One mutation, p.Arg80Gln, had residual enzyme activity (20%) albeit with a much lower reaction velocity than normal and was found to have an impaired ability to bind NADPH.

There is no genotype-phenotype correlation in this disorder with high variability seen even within families with the same *HSD17B3* mutation.

10.4 Diagnosis

The disorder may present with genital ambiguity at birth, inguinal hernias or post-pubertal virilisation. Clinical examination will be needed to establish whether Wolffian duct differentiation and Müllerian duct regression has occurred and to determine whether the testes are present but undescended. As the most common cause of genital ambiguity and virilisation is likely to be congenital adrenal hyperplasia (CAH), it is important to exclude possible adrenal disease by measuring serum cortisol, if necessary post-ACTH stimulation. A normal cortisol response would normally exclude CAH, but in the case of late-onset forms of CAH where residual enzyme activity is present, cortisol may be within the normal range, albeit at the low end, and therefore should be excluded by urine steroid profile. If CAH is excluded one then needs to consider disorders of gonadal steroidogenesis and

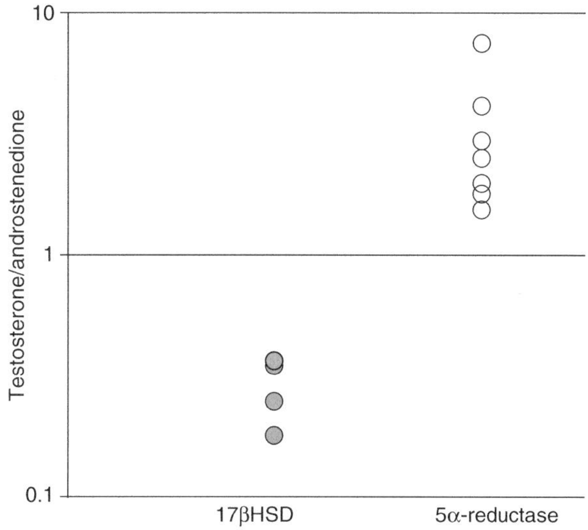

Fig. 10.3 Serum testosterone/androstenedione (nmol/L:nmol/L) ratio in cases of 17βHSD3 and 5α-reductase deficiency with intact gonads

action: 5α-reductase deficiency and androgen receptor defects. Karyotype analysis is important to determine whether virilisation is appropriate for gender.

The primary serum steroid abnormality in 17βHSD3 deficiency is the finding of increased androstenedione relative to testosterone in patients with intact testes. Serum androstenedione concentrations may be as high as 35 nmol/L post puberty, and testosterone can be significant—at the low end of normal for a male. In prepubertal subjects testicular stimulation with human chorionic gonadotrophin will be required prior to measurement of testosterone and androstenedione. Controls typically have a testosterone/androstenedione ratio >1.0, while affected individuals have ratios less than 0.8. By contrast, individuals with 5α-reductase deficiency usually have normal testosterone/androstenedione ratios (Fig. 10.3). Gonadotrophins, in particular luteinising hormone, are typically high after puberty reflecting primary gonadal failure. In those in whom gonadectomy has been performed, genetic testing is really the only reliable way of making a diagnosis.

A urine steroid profile is a useful part of the investigation not to make a direct diagnosis but to exclude 5α-reductase, CAH and adrenal tumours as the cause of virilisation. There are no useful metabolites that can be used to diagnose 17βHSD3 deficiency; the amount of androstenedione produced in this disorder is generally too low to significantly alter the output of urine metabolites although in some cases with intact testes, the adrenal androgens may be elevated relative to cortisol metabolites.

10.5 Case Study

A 16-year-old female presented with primary amenorrhoea, voice deepening and hirsutism. On examination clitoromegaly was noted and she had palpable inguinal gonads and a blind-ending vagina. Prader staging of pubertal development was scored as 0. Her karyotype was 46XY. The differential diagnosis was either 17βHSD3 or 5α-reductase deficiencies or a partial androgen receptor defect. Serum hormone results revealed LH of 24 IU/L, testosterone 5.5 nmol/L and androstenedione 30.1 nmol/L. A defect in the androgen receptor was felt to be unlikely as testosterone was below the normal range for an adult male. The testosterone/androstenedione ratio was 0.18, consistent with 17βHSD3 deficiency, and this was confirmed by the finding of homozygosity for the c.201+1G>A splice site change in *HSD17B3*. A gonadectomy was subsequently performed and oestrogen replacement commenced.

10.6 Steroid Profile

A urine steroid profile from a patient with 17βHSD3 deficiency and intact gonads is shown in Fig. 10.4. There is no particular pattern of steroids seen that are diagnostic for this disorder. The ratio of adrenal androgens to total cortisol metabolites, i.e. (A + Ae)/(THE + THF + 5αTHF), has been mooted as a useful measurement for the diagnosis of 17βHSD3, presumably as one might expect a higher output of androsterone and aetiocholanolone as a result of the raised serum androstenedione. However, in our experience this ratio had no discriminatory value (Fig. 10.5).

The profile is, however, useful to exclude 5α-reductase deficiency using the metabolite pairs 5α-tetrahydrocortisol (5αTHF)/5β-tetrahydrocortisol (THF) and androsterone (5α)/aetiocholanolone (5β) (An/Ae) (Table 10.1) (see Chap. 11). In addition, for those presenting with signs of virilisation, a normal profile would exclude the possibility of an androgen-secreting tumour as well as virilising forms of congenital adrenal hyperplasia. The urine steroid profile can still be

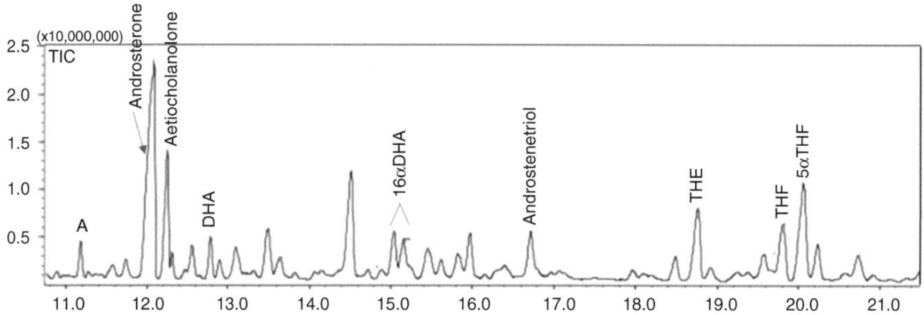

Fig. 10.4 Steroid profile from 46XY female with 17βHSD deficiency and intact gonads showing elevated androsterone compared with aetiocholanolone and increased adrenal androgens to cortisol metabolites. The rest of the profile is unremarkable. The main value of a steroid profile in this disorder is to exclude other potential causes of 46XY DSD

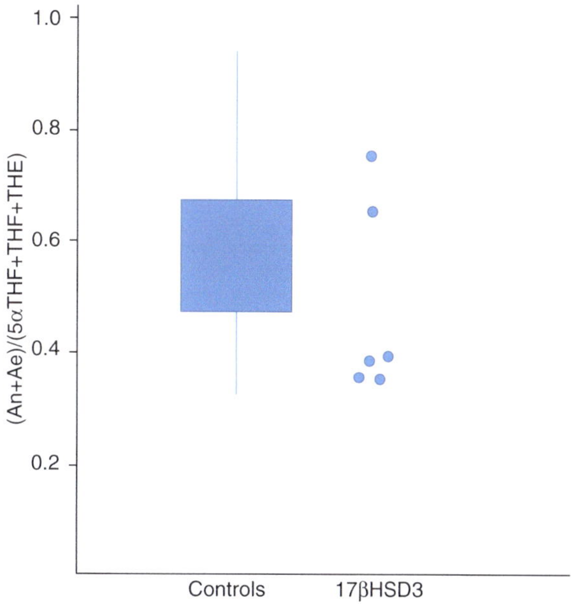

Fig. 10.5 (An/Ae)/(5αTHF + THF + THE) ratio calculated from urine steroid profiles of 17βHSD patients with intact gonads compared with normal male controls

Table 10.1 Steroid metabolites, retention times (methylene units, MU) of their MO-TMS derivatives and characteristic ions (see appendix for spectra)

Steroid	Trivial name	MU	Relevant ions
5α-Androstan-3α-ol-17-one	Androsterone	25.11	270, 360
5β-Androstan-3α-ol-17-one	Aetiocholanolone	25.28	270, 360
5β-Pregnan-3α,17,21-triol-11,20-dione	Tetrahydrocortisone (THE)	29.65	578, 488
5β-Pregnan-3α,11β,17,21-tetrol-20-one	Tetrahydrocortisol (THF)	30.24	652, 472
5α-Pregnan-3α,11β,17,21-tetrol-20-one	alloTHF	30.39	652, 472

used for this purpose even if gonadectomy precedes the biochemical investigation.

10.7 Treatment

As with all DSD the genetic sex, the sex of rearing and degree of virilisation all need to be taken into consideration prior to initiation of treatment. In some cases, gonadectomy will have occurred in childhood, and oestrogen replacement treatment will be required at puberty for those raised as female. Testosterone supplements in the form of oral testosterone undecanoate or as transdermal patches may be needed for incompletely virilised males. Adrenal steroid biosynthesis is completely unaffected so no glucocorticoid or mineralocorticoid replacement is required.

Further Reading

General

Mindnich R, Möller G, Adamski J. The role of 17 beta-hydroxysteroid dehydrogenases. Mol Cell Endocrinol. 2004;218:7–20.

Stukenborg JB, Colón E, Soder Ö. Ontogenesis of testis development and function in humans. Sex Dev. 2010;4:199–212.

Yang Z, Ye L, Wang W, Zhao Y, Wang W, Jia H, Dong Z, Chen Y, Wang W, Ning G, Sun S. 17β-Hydroxysteroid dehydrogenase 3 deficiency: three case reports and a systematic review. J Steroid Biochem Mol Biol. 2017;174:141–5.

Steroid 5α-Reductase Deficiency

11

Gill Rumsby

11.1 Introduction

Androgens play an important role in the development of the male fetus. The Sertoli cells of the fetal testis produce anti-Müllerian hormone (AMH) that prevents development of the Müllerian ducts into the uterus and fallopian tubes. The testicular Leydig cells produce testosterone that is required for development of the seminal vesicle, vas deferens and epididymis, but it is not sufficient for the development of the male external genitalia, i.e. the penis and scrotum, nor for the urethra and a functioning prostate gland. Another androgen, dihydrotestosterone (DHT), is necessary for this stage of development. It is formed from testosterone by reduction across the 4-5 double bond in the steroid A ring in a reaction catalysed by the enzyme 5α-reductase (Fig. 11.1). DHT has approximately two to ten times greater affinity for the androgen receptor than testosterone and dissociates more slowly keeping the androgen receptor in a conformation that is more resistant to degradation.

There are two human 5α-reductase isoenzymes, type 1 (SRD5A1) and type 2 (SRD5A2). A third enzyme (SRD5A3) has also been reported but is a polyprenol reductase and needed for the N-glycosylation of proteins and will not be discussed further. The type 1 and 2 enzymes are hydrophobic, membrane-bound, NADPH-dependent reductases with approximately 50% identity but have different tissue distributions and are encoded by different genes. The type 1 enzyme is not found in fetal tissues but is expressed in the liver and, post puberty, in non-genital skin. The type 2 enzyme is expressed in the fetus and in genital skin, liver and normal prostate. Both enzymes also play a wider role in the metabolism of the steroids progesterone and 17-hydroxyprogesterone as well as cortisol, corticosterone and cortisone. Reduction

G. Rumsby
Department of Clinical Biochemistry, University College London Hospitals, London, UK
e-mail: gill.rumsby@nhs.net

G. Rumsby, G. M. Woodward (eds.), *Disorders of Steroidogenesis*,
https://doi.org/10.1007/978-3-319-96364-8_11

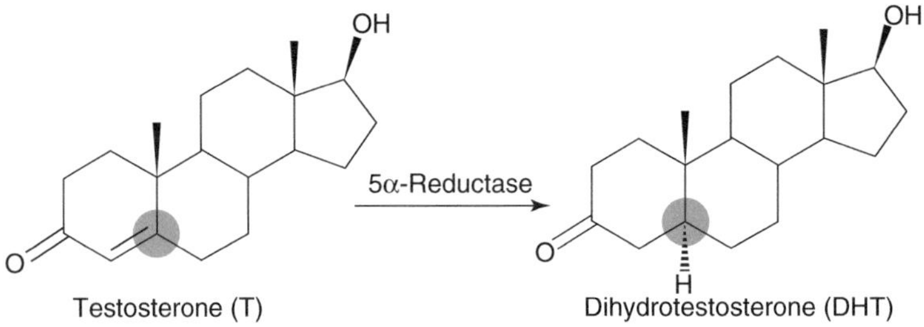

Fig. 11.1 Reaction catalysed by steroid 5α-reductase type 2

at C5 is one of the initial steps in hepatic metabolism of these steroids followed by either further metabolism or conjugation prior to excretion in the urine. The type 1 enzyme is abundantly expressed in the liver, is highly active with C21 steroids and is thought to play the predominant role in hepatic metabolism of steroids. Nevertheless, there is significant suppression of 5-alpha metabolites of C21 steroids in urine in cases of congenital 5α-reductase deficiency, i.e. type 2 enzyme deficiency, emphasising the importance of both isoenzymes in cortisol metabolism.

Suppression of 5α-reductase activity is used as a treatment for prostatic hyperplasia. One of these inhibitors, finasteride, selectively inhibits the type 2 enzyme, whereas another, dutasteride, inhibits both.

11.2 Presentation

The neonatal presentation of 5α-reductase deficiency is usually with a degree of genital ambiguity sufficient to render gender assignment impossible. Thus, the paediatrician is alerted to perform further investigations. An expression of masculinity score (EMS) is made that is based on four clinical features:

1. Presence of gonads in labioscrotal folds
2. Fusion of labioscrotal folds
3. Size of phallus
4. Site of urinary meatus

A score of 12 is found in most normal males; anything less than 11 needs to be further investigated.

In the case of 5α-reductase deficiency, ambiguity may include any or a combination of the following: micropenis, hypospadias, bifid scrotum or single urogenital opening in a phenotypic female. Further investigations revealing the presence of testes would, along with a 46XY karyotype, guide biochemical testing (see diagnosis).

In some cases, the disorder does not manifest until puberty when virilisation occurs in a phenotypic female with 46XY karyotype. This virilisation may be driven by the action of 5α-reductase 1 enzyme on testosterone produced by the pubertal testes now under the stimulation of pituitary gonadotropins, or it could simply reflect the increased concentration of testosterone acting on the androgen receptor at this time. Virilisation causes phallic growth, rugation and pigmentation of the scrotum, increased musculature, voice deepening and hair growth in a male pattern. Not surprisingly, this situation is quite catastrophic for the individual concerned and a rapid diagnosis is required. The first description of this disease in a Dominican Republic kindred found that several individuals subsequently changed their sex from female to male as virilisation occurred. Post puberty it was noted that final height was unimpaired, but there was a noticeable decrease in body hair and lack of hairline recession, the latter subsequently prompting the use of 5α-reductase inhibitors as treatments for male pattern baldness.

The disorder appears to be less problematic in 46XX individuals. In this case the phenotype is associated with decreased body hair, no acne and normal fertility. There has been some suggestion that delayed menarche may be a feature of enzyme deficiency, but the numbers of cases studied are too few to draw any firm conclusions.

11.3 Genetics

The disorder is of autosomal recessive inheritance—the gene encoding the type 2 enzyme, *SRD5A2*, is found on the short arm of chromosome 2 and contains 5 exons spread across 50 kb of genomic DNA. More than 60 mutations have been described—a mix of missense changes, deletions and splice site mutations. The largest numbers of patients come from three self-contained communities in New Guinea, the Dominican Republic and Turkey. The mutation in the first group was found to be a major deletion knocking out most of the gene, while in the second group, a missense change, p.Arg246Trp, was found that affected binding to NADPH. In the Turkish cohort, a single-base deletion, c.753delA, was found in exon 5 leading to a frameshift encoding an additional 23 amino acids at the carboxy-terminal of the protein with the effect of complete loss of enzyme activity. Another missense change affecting amino acid 246, i.e. p.Arg246Gln, is relatively common in patients of Pakistani and Sri Lankan origin suggesting a possible founder effect.

11.4 Diagnosis

Any investigation of the neonate with ambiguous genitalia will be heavily dependent on the chromosomal sex so a karyotype is essential to determine whether the child is an incompletely virilised male or an over virilised female. In the case of 5α-reductase deficiency presenting in a 46XY child with genital ambiguity, the differential diagnosis needs to include other disorders of impaired androgen synthesis and action, i.e. congenital adrenal hyperplasia as a result of 3β-hydroxysteroid dehydrogenase, 17-hydroxylase/17,20-lyase and cytochrome P450 oxidoreductase deficiencies and gonadal steroid disorders including 17β-hydroxysteroid dehydrogenase and 5α-reductase deficiencies, in addition to possible androgen receptor defects. Initial investigations may include the measurement of testosterone and 17-hydroxyprogesterone in the untreated child, but these results may be misleading in the newborn period, particularly if performed by immunoassay as there can be interference from other fetal steroids. Steroid measurements by liquid chromatography-mass spectrometry are preferred for these analyses. If a urine steroid profile and adrenal stimulation with ACTH excludes congenital adrenal hyperplasia, then disorders affecting gonadal steroid synthesis alone need further investigation. In males with intact testes, testosterone synthesis tends to be high at birth falling over the first month before rising again to a peak around day 70 prior to falling again to prepubertal levels. Thus, it may be possible to determine from an unstimulated blood sample whether testosterone synthesis is normal. Otherwise testicular stimulation is required with human chorionic gonadotropin (hCG). This test is either conducted over 3 days or 3 weeks with measurement of testosterone and DHT before and after the test. The 3-day test requires intramuscular injection of 1000–1500 units hCG on 3 consecutive days, while the 3-week test requires an additional administration of 1500 units on 2 days a week for the following 2 weeks. In the presence of normal testicular function, one would expect a response by both testosterone and DHT although the actual cut-offs defining a 'normal' response are unclear and the methodology used can also impact upon the results. The Society for Endocrinology Clinical Guidance for a child with suspected disorder of sex development suggests that a testosterone response post hCG of twice baseline value or above the upper limit of the prepubertal range could be classed as a satisfactory response. In addition a ratio of testosterone/DHT of greater than 30:1 post stimulation would be highly suggestive of 5α-reductase deficiency. In our series of genetically proven paediatric cases, 4 of 11 failed to exceed this ratio after the 3-day hCG stimulation test, with 2 of the 4 subsequently achieving it after the 3-week test. Historically the analytical performance of DHT assays has been poor leading to misdiagnosis. While this situation is now improving with the move to mass-spectrometric assays, there is limited data available to establish diagnostic cut-offs. For this reason, the urine steroid profile is potentially a better test for 5α-reductase deficiency albeit with the caveat that it has limited value in the neonate as there are relatively little 5α and 5β cortisol metabolites excreted before 3 months of age owing to the very active 11β-hydroxysteroid dehydrogenase 2 enzyme that rapidly converts cortisol to cortisone at this time. Genetic testing is therefore useful to confirm 5α-reductase deficiency in a child in whom a normal testosterone response is obtained.

Definitive diagnosis can also be made by the demonstration of decreased 5α-reductase activity in genital skin fibroblasts, but this is a highly specialised technique, not routinely available, and to a large extent is replaced by genetic testing.

Measurement of anti-Müllerian hormone (AMH) is often performed in cases of genital ambiguity. This hormone is produced by the Sertoli cells of the testis and the granulosa cells of the ovary. It is, however, detectable from birth at much higher levels in boys than girls helping to confirm the presence of testicular tissue.

Table 11.1 Reference ranges for various 5α/β pairs of steroids in normal individuals

	An/Ae	5αTHF/THF	αTHB/THB
Males			
<6 years[a]	0.52–3.90	1.10–3.64	2.12–6.58[a]
6–10 years[a]	0.47–5.58	0.43–5.49	0.72–4.83[a]
11–17 years[a]	1.03–2.99	0.73–2.66	0.69–4.20[a]
Males adult[b]	0.67–2.20	0.42–1.1	0.84–3.50[a]
Females adult[b]	0.42–1.08	0.17–0.95	0.88–2.88[a]

[a]Chan et al. (2009)
[b]Berra et al. (2011)

After 3–6 months of age, one can measure the ratio of various 5-alpha/5-beta metabolite pairs, e.g. 5α-tetrahydrocortisol/tetrahydrocortisol (5αTHF/THF), 5α-tetrahydrocorticosterone/tetrahydrocorticosterone (αTHB/THB) and, following adrenarche, the additional androsterone/aetiocholanolone (An/Ae) pair. In our experience, An/Ae and 5αTHF/THF ratios have proved the most satisfactory. An/Ae was 100% sensitive with a specificity of 83%, while 5αTHF/THF pairing was 90% sensitive with 69% specificity. Table 11.1 shows typical results for these ratios in normal individuals. Younger children tend to have a higher excretion of 5-alpha steroids accounting for the slightly higher ratio in the younger age groups.

Individuals may also present later in their teenage years and beyond with virilisation of an apparent female and failure to menstruate. This virilisation is driven by testicular-derived testosterone for those still with intact testes. Investigation again requires karyotype analysis, serum androgen measurements and a urine steroid profile, the latter enabling the investigation of all forms of virilising congenital adrenal hyperplasia, 5α-reductase deficiency and virilising tumours simultaneously. Some may have had earlier gonadectomies, possibly after presenting with inguinal hernias, and will thus present with delayed puberty. If gonadectomy has already occurred in childhood without a diagnosis being made, the urine steroid profile is invaluable as testicular androgen is no longer present and thus serum hormone studies are unhelpful (Fig. 11.2).

A variety of other conditions can affect the relative activity of 5α- to 5β-reductase. There is a diurnal variation with highest ratios achieved in the second half of the day. Thyroxine appears to have a direct stimulatory effect on 5α-reductase activity, and both the An/Ae and 5αTHF/THF ratios are increased in hyperthyroidism by as much as twofold normal. Conversely, profound hypothyroidism can give a similar urine steroid profile to 5α-reductase deficiency affecting both C19 and C21 metabolite pairs, and this must be excluded by the measurement of the thyroid hormones TSH and free thyroxine. Chronic hypercortisolism, i.e. Cushing's syndrome, shows a decreased conversion of C21 steroids to 5α-reduced metabolites, but a lesser affect is seen on the C19 steroids (see Chap. 16). Adipose tissue contains 5α- but not 5β-reductase; consequently ratios can be elevated in obesity reflecting the increased tissue mass. Anorexia nervosa on the other hand can lead to a marked reduction in the 5α/5β ratio. Polycystic ovarian syndrome has been shown by some to have

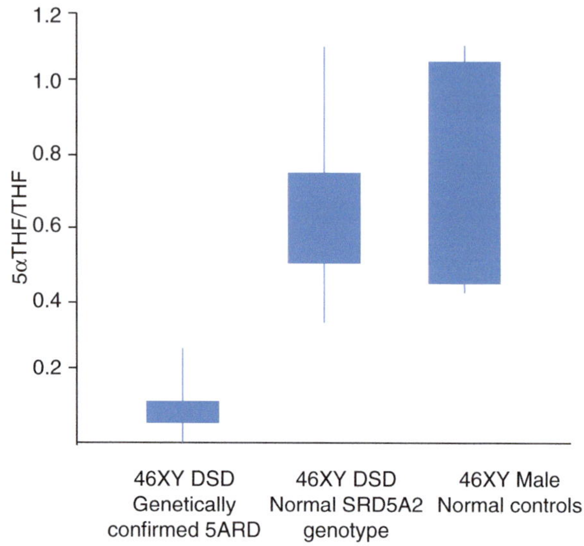

Fig. 11.2 Ratio of 5αTHF/THF in adult patients with 46XY DSD caused by genetically confirmed 5α-reductase deficiency (5ARD), other cases of 46XY DSD in whom 5ARD has been excluded and normal controls. Boxes show 25th and 95th percentiles, and whiskers range

elevated 5α/5β ratio of both C21 and C19 steroids, but this finding is by no means diagnostic of this disorder and disputed by others. There is some evidence for insulin as a stimulant of 5α-reductase activity.

In some of these secondary cases we do not always know if the effect is on the 5α- or the 5β-reductase enzyme. A complete deficiency of 5β-reductase has been described that leads to an exceptionally high ratio of 5αTHF/THF, greater than 300 and An/Ae of greater than 6. This congenital disorder, which has a cholestatic phenotype, is due to a defect in the aldo-ketoreductase type 1 (AKRID1) enzyme and leads to bile acid insufficiency.

11.5 Case Study

11.5.1 Neonatal Case Study

Following a full-term pregnancy and normal delivery, ambiguous genitalia (severe hypospadias) were noted at 5 weeks of age. The child was referred to a paediatric endocrinologist at 5 months of age. Ultrasound showed bilateral testes and no uterus or ovaries. A single perineal opening with bilateral swellings in labioscrotal folds, subsequently shown to be testes, was noted. Examination under anaesthesia confirmed bilateral descended testes, an underdeveloped scrotum and extremely small penis. A 3-day HCG test was performed in which human chorionic gonadotropin was administered to the child and samples taken for testosterone and dihydrotestosterone (DHT) prior to hCG and 3 days later. The results are shown in Table 11.2.

DHT is normally approximately one-tenth the concentration of testosterone. At low testosterone concentrations, the test is of limited use, and the urine steroid

Table 11.2 Response of testosterone and DHT to hCG stimulation test in a child with possible 5α-reductase deficiency

Time	Testosterone (nmol/L)	Dihydrotestosterone (nmol/L)
0	<0.41	<0.27
3 days	13.7	0.37

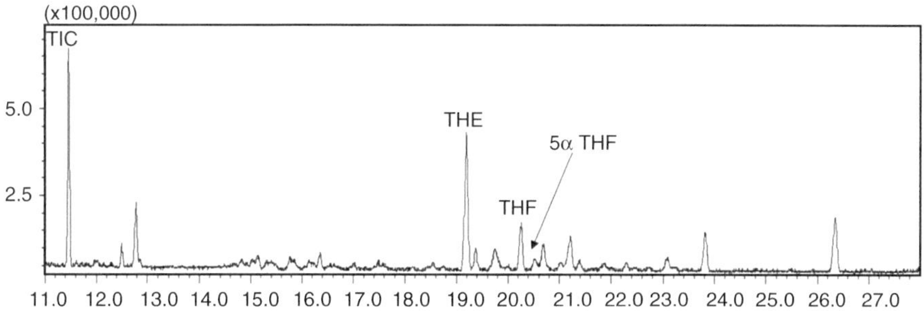

Fig. 11.3 Urine steroid profile from a 1-year-old child with 5α-reductase deficiency. At this age there is only one set of metabolites from which to make the diagnosis: 5αTHF/THF

profile is of more value. In this particular case, the results showed an adequate response of testosterone to the hCG challenge, but DHT synthesis was significantly impaired suggestive of 5α-reductase deficiency. The urine steroid profile (Fig. 11.3) had undetectable 5-alpha-reduced cortisol metabolite, 5αTHF, leading to a markedly decreased 5α/5β ratio (5αTHF/THF = <0.1, normal 1.10–3.64). At this age, i.e. prior to adrenarche, this is the only useful metabolite pair as the adrenal androgens, An/Ae, are not present in significant amounts to aid diagnosis.

Subsequent genetic testing found homozygosity for a variant, c.100G>A, that caused a missense change, p.(Gly34Arg)—a known pathological mutation—confirming a diagnosis of 5ARD.

11.5.2 Late Presentation

A female presented age 16 with primary amenorrhoea and voice deepening. Testes were found on ultrasound examination and were removed age 18 years without a diagnosis being made. She presented to the adult Disorders of Sex development clinic age 23 years. On examination, she was found to have clitoromegaly with a single perineal opening and no uterus (Prader stage between 1 and 2). The differential diagnosis included 17-hydroxylase deficiency, 17β-hydroxysteroid dehydrogenase deficiency, 5ARD and androgen receptor defects. In the absence of testes serum androgens, including androstenedione, testosterone and DHT would be uninformative. The urine steroid profile showed a characteristic decrease in 5α metabolites: An/Ae 0.19 (reference range 0.67–2.20) and 5αTHF/THF 0.20 (reference range 0.42–1.10). Genetic testing confirmed the diagnosis of 5α-reductase deficiency in this patient finding homozygosity for c.737G>A encoding the known pathological missense mutation, p.Arg246Gln.

11.6 Steroid Profile

The retention times of the components of the various 5α/5β steroid pairs are shown in Table 11.3.

The finding of markedly decreased 5-alpha-reduced metabolites is consistent with 5α-reductase deficiency (Figs. 11.3 and 11.4), but, as mentioned earlier, this can be inherited or secondary to other disorders or drug treatments (see below). In the first 3 months of life, cortisol is rapidly converted to cortisone, and therefore there is little THF and 5αTHF present although it may still be possible to pick these up using selective ion monitoring at *m/z* 652 (M^+−31). A typical steroid profile from a 5-month-old child with 5α-reductase deficiency is shown in Fig. 11.3, where diagnosis was based on the decreased 5αTHF/THF ratio. There are no adrenal

Table 11.3 Pairs of steroids analysed for the diagnosis of 5α-reductase deficiency, retention times (methylene units, MU) of their MO-TMS derivatives and characteristic ions (see appendix for spectra)

Steroid	Trivial name	MU	Ions
5α-Androstan-3α-ol-17-one	Androsterone (5α)	25.11	270, 360
5β-Androstan-3α-ol-17-one	Aetiocholanolone (5β)	25.28	270, 360
5β-Pregnan-3α,11β,21-triol-20-one	Tetrahydrocorticosterone (5β)	30.00/30.16	564, 188
5α-Pregnan-3α,11β,21-triol-20-one	Allo-tetrahydrocorticosterone (5α)	30.16/30.80	564, 188
5β-Pregnan-3α,11β,17,21-tetrol-20-one	Tetrahydrocortisol (THF) (5β)	30.24	652, 472
5α-Pregnan-3α,11β,17,21-tetrol-20-one	Allo-tetrahydrocortisol (alloTHF) (5α)	30.39	652, 472

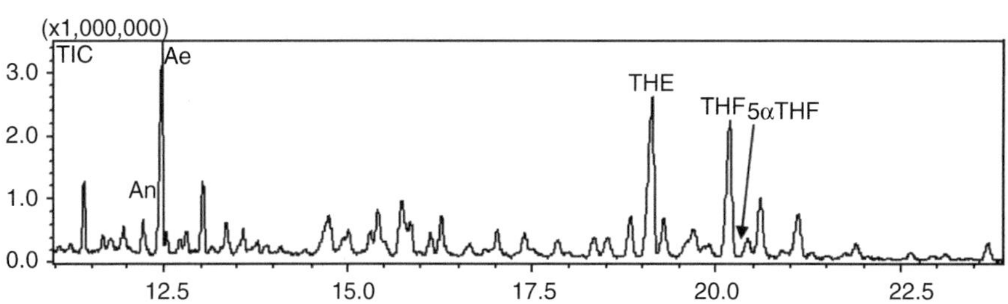

Fig. 11.4 It shows the situation in teenager where both pairs of metabolites, An/Ae and 5αTHF/THF, can be used for diagnosis. The 5α metabolites are not completely suppressed, the residual activity accounted for by the 5α-reductase 1 enzyme

androgens present at this time, and so the cortisol metabolites are the only pair that can be used for diagnosis.

Some drug treatments can give a false-positive diagnosis of 5α-reductase deficiency. The inhibitors finasteride and dutasteride are used for treatment of prostate hypertrophy and prostate cancer and thus might be expected to crop up in the older male patient. Finasteride has also found a role in the treatment of male pattern baldness so its use may be more prevalent than before in younger men. Dutasteride inhibits both type 1 and type 2 enzymes so will be more obviously an artefact. Mitotane, a powerful adrenolytic used for the treatment of adrenal tumours, also causes a marked reduction in 5α/5β ratio of both C19 and C21 steroids.

11.7 Treatment

If a male sex of rearing is favoured, dihydrotestosterone can be given to enhance penile growth and can be administered by use of DHT gel. Testosterone supplementation is not suitable. Surgery may be required to repair hypospadias and orchiopexy to correct cryptorchidism. In those with 46XY genotype, raised as female and presenting with symptoms later in life, psychological counselling is required as the desired course of action may be to continue as a female or to adopt their genetic sex. In the former situation gonadectomy would be required to prevent the virilising effects of testosterone while in the latter additional hormonal and surgical treatment will be required as well as genital surgery.

Further Reading

Diagnosis

Ahmed SF, Achermann JC, Arlt W, et al. UK guidance on the initial evaluation of an infant or an adolescent with a suspected disorder of sex development. Clin Endocrinol. 2011;75:12–26.

Berra M, Williams EL, Muroni B, Creighton SM, Honour JW, Rumsby G, Conway G. Recognition of 5α-reductase 2 deficiency in an adult female 46XY DSD clinic. Eur J Endocrinol. 2011;164:1019–25.

Chan AOK, But BWM, Lau GTC, Lam ALN, Ng KL, et al. Diagnosis of 5alpha-reductase deficiency: a local experience. Hong Kong Med J. 2009;15:130–5.

11β-Hydroxysteroid Dehydrogenase Deficiency

12

Gary M. Woodward

12.1 Introduction

In order to gain a clinical appreciation for 11β-HSD deficiency, an understanding of normal cortisol (F) metabolism is vital. In simple terms, cortisol is "deactivated" by its conversion to cortisone (E) but can also be regenerated by the reverse reaction. The reversible interconversion of cortisol to cortisone is catalysed by 11β-hydroxysteroid dehydrogenase (11β-HSD) (Fig. 12.1) that occurs as two distinct isoforms, 11β-HSD1 and 11β-HSD2, with only 21% identity in coding sequence. The 11β-HSD1 enzyme is ubiquitous but is found predominantly in the liver and adipose tissue and can also be induced in other tissues, while 11β-HSD2 is found in the placenta and kidney and other mineralocorticoid-sensitive tissues such as the colon and salivary glands.

The 11β-HSD1 enzyme is found in the endoplasmic reticulum of the cell. It is a homodimer, attached to the membrane by an N-terminal anchor, and is bidirectional in tissue homogenates but acts predominantly as a cortisone reductase, a reaction favoured by the higher ratio of NADPH to NADP cofactor in the endoplasmic reticulum. The NADPH in turn is generated by hexose-6-phosphate dehydrogenase (H6PDH) which metabolises glucose-6-phosphate to 6-phosphogluconolactone.

The clearance of cortisol and the hypothalamic-pituitary-adrenal (HPA) axis are closely linked. An increase in metabolism and clearance of cortisol are offset by an increase in HPA drive. This ultimately results in an increase in adrenal cortisol production with the aim of maintaining circulating concentrations. Likewise, a decrease in metabolism results in a decrease in HPA drive and less cortisol in the circulation. The conversion of cortisone to cortisol contributes to overall glucocorticoid

G. M. Woodward
Department of Clinical Biochemistry, University College London Hospitals, London, UK
e-mail: Gary.Woodward1@nhs.net

G. Rumsby, G. M. Woodward (eds.), *Disorders of Steroidogenesis*,
https://doi.org/10.1007/978-3-319-96364-8_12

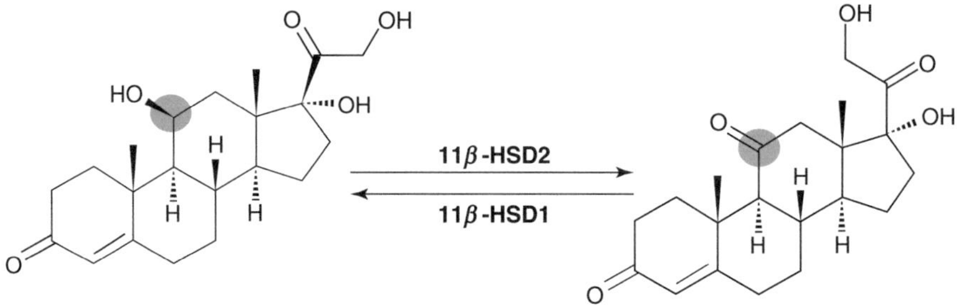

Fig. 12.1 Interconversion of cortisol and cortisone is catalysed by 11β-HSD1 and 11β-HSD2

synthesis and in the absence of 11β-HSD1 leads to lifting of the negative feedback and stimulation of the HPA with increased ACTH release. The reaction is also important for the conversion of some steroids to their active form, e.g. prednisone to prednisolone. Physiologically, there is very limited 11β-HSD1 expression in the first 2–3 months of life, and it is all but absent in fetal tissue. Expression gradually rises in the first year when it reaches adult levels. Levels of active glucocorticoid depend not only on circulating concentrations but also on site-specific activation by tissue-specific cortisone metabolism. Given the activity and tissue expression (liver and adipose) of 11β-HSD1, the enzyme is thought to play a role in obesity, insulin resistance and polycystic ovary syndrome.

The first cases of apparent cortisone reductase deficiency in patients with increased cortisol clearance and adrenal hyperandrogenism had no defect in 11β-HSD1 but were found to be caused by mutations in H6PDH. The effect of these mutations on NADPH availability possibly increased the dehydrogenase activity of 11β-HSD1 and, in conjunction with 11β-HSD2, led to an overall increase in the metabolism and clearance of cortisol. Subsequently individuals have been described with a milder form of cortisone reductase deficiency who were heterozygous for mutations in 11β-HSD1. There is in vitro evidence that these mutants have a dominant-negative effect leading to reduced enzyme activity.

The 11β-HSD2 enzyme is an NAD-dependent dehydrogenase that catalyses the conversion of 11-hydroxylated steroids to the less biologically active 11-oxo steroids. These steroid substrates include cortisol and corticosterone but not aldosterone or dexamethasone. The mineralocorticoid receptor has a similar affinity for cortisol and aldosterone, and therefore the presence of 11β-HSD2 in tissues expressing this receptor serves to protect it from glucocorticoid excess. In the placenta, the enzyme prevents exposure of the fetus to maternal glucocorticoid. The enzyme is also particularly active in the neonate where more than 90% of corticosteroid metabolites have been reported to have an 11-oxo group, and this is illustrated by the presence of predominantly cortisone metabolites with minimal cortisol metabolites in neonatal urine. 11β-HSD2 activity has a direct influence on circulating corticosteroid levels which plays a role in modulating blood pressure. In addition, there are some suggestions that vascular smooth muscle cell 11β-HSD activity changes affect active glucocorticoid concentration and represent an additional factor for underlying hypertension.

Deficiency of 11β-HSD2 results in increased exposure of the renal receptor to cortisol that may then act as a potent mineralocorticoid and increase renal sodium reabsorption. This state can be either inherited or acquired. The inherited form is referred to as apparent mineralocorticoid deficiency (AME) and is characterised by severe, early-onset, low renin hypertension with similarities to mineralocorticoid excess but with suppressed aldosterone. A milder variant of this (AME type 2) has been described in which the enzyme activity is attenuated, but not completely deficient.

Acquired 11β-HSD2 deficiency can arise from excessive liquorice ingestion, Cushing's syndrome, excessive progesterone in pregnancy and renal and liver disease.

Liquorice: The active ingredients in liquorice, glycyrrhetinic acid and glycyrrhizic acid, are competitive inhibitors of 11β-HSD2. Indeed, since the 1940s it has been known that patients who consume large amounts of liquorice may develop hypertension and hypokalaemia, in some cases severe enough to cause cardiac arrhythmia and myopathy. In these cases, both plasma renin activity and aldosterone are suppressed. Like glycyrrhetinic acid, several xenobiotic substances, particularly some plant-derived flavonoids such as naringin, found in grapefruit, exhibit some inhibitory effects on 11β-HSD2. These xenobiotics increase the free cortisol to cortisone ratio, reduce plasma renin activity and cause mild hypokalaemia in some studies.

Cushing's syndrome: The hypertension associated with Cushing's syndrome, particularly in cases of ectopic ACTH production, is characterised by excess mineralocorticoid activity and hypokalaemic alkalosis. It is thought that an increased production of deoxycorticosterone contributes to these clinical features and correlates with the degree of mineralocorticoid excess. ACTH does not directly affect 11β-HSD2; however saturation of the enzyme may occur via ACTH-dependent 11β-HSD2 substrates (i.e. cortisol and corticosterone). As a result the (tetrahydrocortisol + 5α-tetrahydrocortisol)/tetrahydrocortisone (THF + 5αTHF/THE) and free cortisol/cortisone ratios are elevated.

Renal and liver disease: Since 11β-HSD2 is found mainly in the kidney, it is the major site for cortisol to cortisone metabolism. As such, renal disease influences the rate of metabolism and prolongs the circulating cortisol half-life by about 45 min. It should be noted that some steroid medications, such as prednisolone, are also substrates for 11β-HSD2 metabolism. Therefore, renal disease may also increase the half-life of these drugs. Dexamethasone is less affected.

While plasma cortisone concentrations are reduced in renal disease patients with an inverse relationship between cortisone and creatinine levels, negative feedback mechanisms help modulate these effects to ensure plasma cortisol concentrations are unchanged.

In the case of liver disease, severe cases resulting in increased bile acid circulation cause an increased (THF + 5αTHF):THE ratio via inhibition of 11β-HSD2 activity.

Pregnancy: Placental tissue possesses high levels of 11β-HSD2 and is thought to protect the fetus from glucocorticoid exposure. Impaired 11β-HSD2 activity in this tissue is thought to cause intrauterine growth restriction leading to hypertension later in life. High levels of progesterone during pregnancy may lead to inhibition of placental 11β-HSD2 causing pregnancy-induced hypertension and preeclampsia.

Other drugs: There is evidence for inhibition of 11β-HSD2 by the triazole antifungal drugs, posaconazole and itraconazole, based on AME-like symptoms and elevated serum cortisol/cortisone ratios.

12.2 Presentation

11β-HSD1 deficiency is a rare cause of ACTH-driven, adrenal hyperandrogenism in adolescent or young adult females or pseudoprecocious puberty. Symptoms in females include hirsutism, oligomenorrhoea and infertility. Polycystic ovaries may also be present.

Overt 11β-HSD2 deficiency is also extremely rare, but its presentation may be striking. Patients present early in life, usually with low birth weight, muscle weakness, failure to thrive and severe hypertension, possibly with concurrent hypokalaemia and associated metabolic alkalosis and are potentially fatal. Renal insufficiency has also been described in some cases with nephropathies, including nephrocalcinosis and nephrogenic diabetes insipidus. As a result of the severe hypertension, cardiac abnormalities may develop, such as left ventricular hypertrophy and cardiomegaly. These cardiac complications represent the major cause of mortality in these patients due to infarction, stroke and cerebral haemorrhage. Microvascular complications, including hypertensive retinopathy, may also occur. Milder phenotypes present in childhood and in adults with less severe biochemical and clinical features that may include mineralocorticoid-associated hypertension, plasma volume expansion and hypokalaemia.

12.3 Genetics

The *HSD11B1* gene encoding 11β-HSD1 is found on chromosome 1q32.2, but most reported cases of apparent cortisone reductase deficiency are caused by mutations in the *H6PDH* gene, the latter having a more severe phenotype. The disorder is inherited as an autosomal recessive disease, but two cases with biochemically mild cortisone reductase deficiency were identified who had normal *H6PDH* gene sequence but were only heterozygous for variants in *HSD11B1* that abolished or significantly reduced enzyme activity by interfering with protein folding or dimer formation. To explain the disease in these heterozygous cases, it was suggested (and experimentally confirmed) that the formation of heterodimers (mutant protein plus normal protein) led to impaired activity of the enzyme, i.e. a dominant-negative effect.

HSD11B2, encoding 11β-HSD2, is on the long arm of chromosome 16 (16q22) and shares only 20% sequence homology with *HSD11B1*. The gene has 5 exons, and at least 40 mutations, a mixture of missense, nonsense, splice site changes and insertion-deletions, have been reported some affecting the cofactor and/or substrate-binding site and others the dimer interface. Mutations have also now been described in the milder form of the disease, the so-called type 2 variant showing that this is in fact a continuum and not a separate disorder. One of these p.Leu376Pro was found to have approximately 10% of wild-type activity in vitro, and this residual activity possibly accounted for the later presentation. Another change associated with late onset disease is p.Pro227Leu that possibly disrupts the substrate-binding site. There appears to be a poor correlation of genotype with phenotype suggesting that other factors, including dietary salt intake, may influence the phenotype.

12.4 Diagnosis

The diagnosis of 11β-HSD1 includes the differential of causes of hyperandrogenism. Initial investigations will include routine tests including testosterone, sex hormone-binding globulin and androstenedione. If imaging identifies adrenal hypertrophy, then urine steroid profile should be requested to exclude other, more common, causes of adrenal androgen production including 21-hydroxylase and 11-hydroxylase deficiencies in addition to the exclusion of possible adrenal tumour and will have the added advantage of also identifying 11β-HSD1 deficiency. Further confirmation of this disorder requires the administration of 25 mg oral cortisone and the measurement of plasma cortisol and cortisone over a 2.5 h period. In the case of 11HSD1 deficiency, cortisol gives an attenuated response with little response over the first 60 min compared to a control.

Investigation of early-onset hypertension, including possible 11β-HSD2 deficiency, requires measurement of plasma renin and aldosterone. Once it is identified as a low renin hypertension, the source of mineralocorticoid excess needs to be identified. In this case, a urine steroid profile would be an appropriate test as it can confirm/exclude the presence of hypertensive forms of congenital adrenal hyperplasia such as 11- and 17α-hydroxylase deficiencies and exclude Cushing's syndrome by measurement of total cortisol metabolites, as well as review the ratio of cortisol/cortisone metabolites to make a biochemical diagnosis of AME. In AME, ratios of (THF + 5αTHF)/THE of 6.7–33 have been reported with a value of 3.0 in a mild, genetically confirmed case compared with a normal ratio of 0.7–1.1.

12.5 Case Study

A 2-year-old female with birth weight 2.0 kg following a full-term pregnancy had a history of poor weight gain during the first year. She developed muscle weakness age 3 years and was found to have serum sodium of 142 mmol/L and potassium 2.0 mmol/L. She was hypertensive with blood pressure of 160/110 mmHg. Renin and aldosterone were both undetectable. A urine was sent for a steroid profile to exclude hypertensive forms of congenital adrenal hyperplasia, and this was found to have an elevated (THF + 5αTHF)/THE ratio of >40 (reference range 0.7–1.1) consistent with a diagnosis of AME. The 5αTHF/THF ratio was also elevated at 3 (reference range 0.17–0.95) No other abnormal metabolites were present.

12.6 Steroid Profile

Both 11β-HSD1 and 11β-HSD2 are characterised by abnormal ratios of cortisol/cortisone metabolites; the two disorders are, biochemically, mirror images of each other (Table 12.1).

In the case of 11β-HSD1 deficiency, the profile is characterised by an increase in cortisone to cortisol metabolites such that the (5αTHF + THF)/THE ratio is significantly reduced; values less than 0.05 have been reported (reference range males 0.7–1.1) (Fig. 12.2). The ratio of 5αTHF/THF is also lowered suggestive of enhanced

Table 12.1 Steroid metabolites used for assessment of 11β-HSD activity, retention times (methylene units, MU) of their MO-TMS derivatives and characteristic ions (see appendix for spectra)

Steroid	Trivial name	MU	Ions
5β-Pregnan-3α,17,21-triol-11,20-dione	THE	29.69	578, 488
5β-Pregnan-3α,11β,17,21-tetrol-20-one	Tetrahydrocortisol (THF)	30.24	652, 472
5α-Pregnan-3α,11β,17,21-tetrol-20-one	Allo-tetrahydrocortisol (5αTHF)	30.39	652, 472

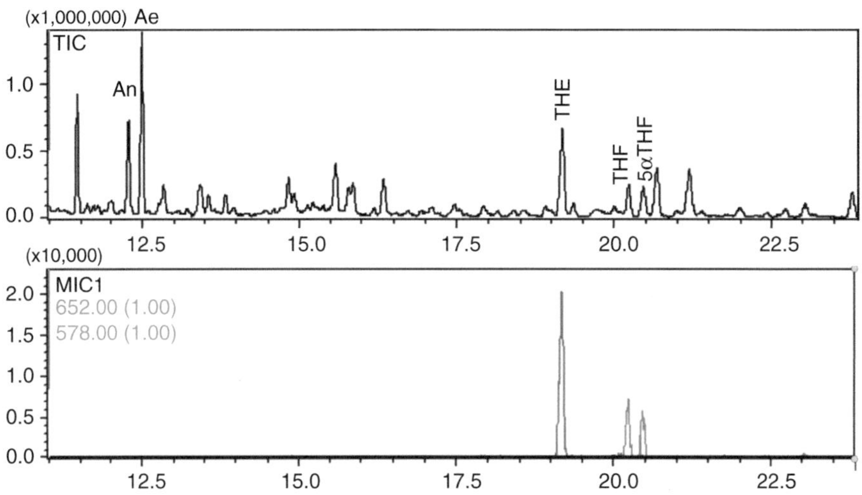

Fig. 12.2 Urine steroid profile from a patient with suspected 11β-HSD1 (cortisone reductase) deficiency. Total ion chromatogram is shown at the top. Note increased output of adrenal androgens androsterone (An) and aetiocholanolone (Ae). The lower chromatogram shows selective ion monitoring for THE (578), THF and 5αTHF (652). Complete deficiency is not present

5β-reductase activity. The effect on adrenal androgens is less clear-cut, in some cases marked elevations of androsterone and aetiocholanolone have been reported, whereas in others these may be within the reference range.

In contrast, urinary steroid metabolite profiles in 11β-HSD2 are characterised by a high excretion of 11β-hydroxycortisol metabolites (THF and cortols) and low excretion of 11-oxo-metabolites (THE and cortolones) (Fig. 12.3). The ratio of (5αTHF + THF)/THE is thus enhanced with values in the order of 6 to greater than 70 reported in the literature. Serum and urinary free cortisol to free cortisone ratios are also elevated. Typically, free cortisone (E) is excreted at a level two to three times that of cortisol (F), while in cases of 11β-HSD2 deficiency levels of free cortisone may be undetectable. A direct measure of urinary free cortisol to free cortisone may better reflect direct renal 11β-HSD2 activity, since THF, 5α-THF and THE are liver-reduced metabolites and reflect both 11β-HSD1 and 11β-HSD2 activity.

The ratio of 5αTHF/THF is increased in 11β-HSD2 deficiency to approximately twice normal, believed to be the result of a reduction in 5β-reductase activity. The underlying reason for the changes in 5β-reductase activity in the two disorders is unknown.

It is important to note that although AME patients have an increased cortisol to cortisone ratio with an apparent increased free cortisol half-life, they do not exhibit features of Cushing's owing to an intact negative feedback mechanism that maintains normal levels of circulating cortisol.

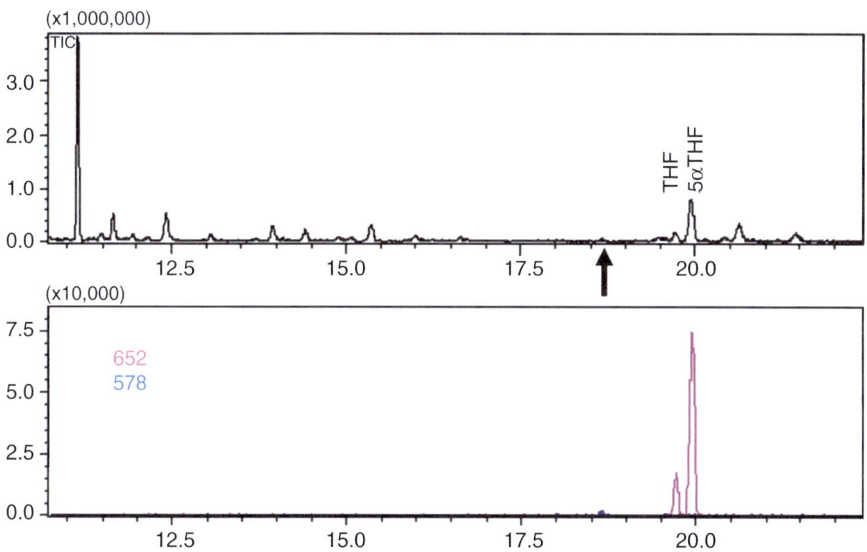

Fig. 12.3 Urine steroid profile from patient with 11β-HSD2 deficiency. Total ion chromatogram is shown at the top and selective ion chromatogram to detect THE (578), THF and 5αTHF (652) at the bottom. The arrow shows the expected position of THE

12.7 Treatment

Little information is available on treatment for 11β-HSD1. The HPA axis can be suppressed by dexamethasone but this is at the risk of glucocorticoid excess.

For 11β-HSD2, initial therapy will be directed at correcting the potentially life-threatening disturbances such as hypokalaemia and severe hypertension. Dexamethasone administration can be used to suppress cortisol production and is effective in some, but not all, cases. Additional antihypertensive medications and diuretics (such as amiloride, triamterene and thiazides) are also used. Spironolactone acts as a mineralocorticoid receptor antagonist and may be beneficial but has to be used at high doses. In cases of unresponsive hypertension, renal transplant has been reported as a curative treatment for this condition in at least one case.

Further Reading

Wider Role of 11β-HSD1

Cooper MS, Stewart PM. 11β-Hydroxysteroid dehydrogenase type 1 and its role in the hypothalamic-pituitary-adrenal axis, metabolic syndrome and inflammation. J Clin Endocrinol Metab. 2009;94:4645–54.

Bailey MA. 11β-Hydroxysteroid dehydrogenases and hypertension in the metabolic syndrome. Curr Hypertens Rep. 2017;19:100.

Update on Genetics and Biochemistry of 11β-HSD2

Yau M, Haider S, Khattab A, et al. Clinical, genetic, and structural basis of apparent mineralocorticoid excess due to 11β-hydroxysteroid dehydrogenase type 2 deficiency. Proc Natl Acad Sci U S A. 2017;114(52):E11248–56.

Steroid Sulphotransferase and Sulphatase Deficiency

13

Gill Rumsby

13.1 Introduction

The process of conjugation of steroid molecules makes them water soluble and enables their excretion via the renal tract. It also has the effect of making them less reactive by reducing their affinity for steroid receptors although in some cases, e.g. dehydroepiandrosterone sulphate (DHEAS) and pregnenolone sulphate, the sulphated steroid can act as a neuromodulator in its own right. Sulphation increases the half-life of the hormone and provides a reservoir of sulphated steroids with regeneration into active steroids in tissues containing the relevant deconjugating enzymes (Fig. 13.1). Sulphation is also required for the phase II detoxification of xenobiotics and to maintain structure and function of tissues as, for example, in the case of the glycosaminoglycans that are components of connective tissues.

Sulphation occurs by the addition of a sulphonate (SO_3^{2-}) group to one or more hydroxyl moieties on the steroid molecule. Sulphate is mainly obtained from dietary intake with a minor amount from the sulphur-containing amino acids, methionine and cysteine. Methionine is converted to cysteine by the transsulphuration pathway, followed by oxidation of cysteine to sulphate (SO_4^{2-}). Dietary sulphate is actively absorbed into the circulation via the small intestine and taken up by cells through tissue-specific transporters. The kidney plays an active role in maintaining the circulating concentration of sulphate at approx. 0.3 mmol/L. Following filtration by the renal glomerulus, sulphate is reabsorbed by the proximal tubular cells with less than 26% excreted in urine. Reabsorption takes place via two solute transporter carrier (SLC) membrane transporters, one on the apical membrane and one on the basolateral membrane. The apical membrane transporter, SLC13A1, is a Na^+-dependent sulphate transporter and defects in this transporter lead to renal sulphate

G. Rumsby
Department of Clinical Biochemistry, University College London Hospitals, London, UK
e-mail: gill.rumsby@nhs.net

G. Rumsby, G. M. Woodward (eds.), *Disorders of Steroidogenesis*,
https://doi.org/10.1007/978-3-319-96364-8_13

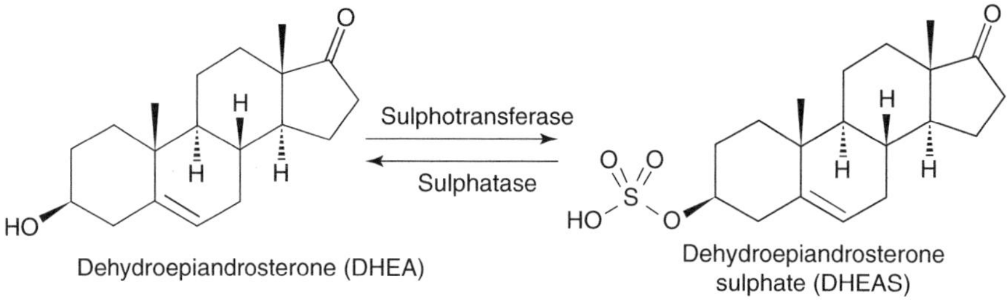

Fig. 13.1 Interconversion of DHEA and DHEAS

Table 13.1 Steroid sulphotransferases (SULT) and their primary substrates

SULT	Primary steroid substrate	Chromosomal location of gene
SULT2A1 SULT1E1	DHEA	19q13.3 4q13.1
SULT2A1	Androsterone	19q13.3
SULT2A1 SULT2B1a	Pregnenolone	19q13.3 19q13.3
SULT1E1	Oestrone	4q13.1
SULT1E1 SULT1A1	Oestradiol	4q13.1 16p12.1
SULT2B1b	Cholesterol	19q13.3

loss. The basolateral membrane transporter, SLC26A1, is an anion exchanger that mediates electroneutral exchange of sulphate-oxalate, sulphate-bicarbonate and oxalate-bicarbonate. Sulphate can also be generated intracellularly by the action of sulphatase enzymes located in the lysosomes.

The mechanism of sulphation requires the presence of the universal sulphonate donor, 5′-phosphoadenosine-3′-phosphosulphate (PAPS), that is synthesised from ATP in two steps catalysed by the enzyme PAPS synthase 2 (PAPSS2). Firstly, there is sulphurylation of ATP to form adenosine-5′-phosphosulphate followed by phosphorylation to form PAPS. The reaction by-product, 3′-phosphoadenosine-5′-phosphate (PAP), is degraded by specific phosphatases to AMP and phosphate. There are at least 62 sulphotransferase genes of which 13 encode sulphotransferase enzymes in the cytosol (SULTs) that conjugate steroids, thyroid hormones, bile acids, neurotransmitters and xenobiotics. The remainder are membrane-bound enzymes in the Golgi apparatus that mediate the sulphonation of proteoglycans and lipids. This latter group will not be discussed further in this chapter. There are five SULTs that actively conjugate steroids. These enzymes and their substrates are shown in Table 13.1. There is considerable overlap in substrate specificity and thus other enzymes may be able to compensate in deficiency states.

Circulating sulphonated steroids require the assistance of organic acid transporter polypeptides (OATPs) to enter cells where they can be deconjugated to active steroids. OATPs are widely expressed and mediate the cellular uptake of a wide number of metabolites including steroids and xenobiotics. The transporters are bidirectional but likely to be more involved with influx; they operate independently of sodium and ATP, but it is not yet clear whether this is an electroneutral process in exchange for ions such as bicarbonate. There is also evidence for the involvement of the ATP-binding cassette transporters, MRP1 and MRP4, in the efflux of DHEAS and oestrone sulphate from the cell.

The SULT enzymes are predominantly expressed in the colon, kidney, brain and adrenal gland. SULT2A1 enzyme is located in the zona reticularis of the adrenal gland and is therefore responsible for the high output of DHEAS from this gland. The substrates of this enzyme include pregnenolone and 17α-hydroxypregnenolone as well as DHEA. Once in the sulphate form, these steroids are no longer available as substrates for 3β-hydroxysteroid dehydrogenase and therefore prevent their use in the mineralocorticoid and glucocorticoid pathways. However, as these sulphated steroids are also poor substrates for the 17α-hydroxylase enzyme, cells synthesising DHEA would also require high expression of steroid sulphatase to activate the substrates. There is considerable variation in DHEAS production throughout life. The human fetal adrenal produces high levels of SULT2A1 in the fetal zone cells but none is seen in the neocortex. After birth and involution of the fetal zone, there is little expression of SULT2A1 until the onset of adrenarche after which it increases in the expanding zona reticularis. DHEAS continues to be expressed throughout life although serum levels fall in later life by 70% of maximum.

The sulphatase enzymes cleave the sulphate moiety restoring the steroid hormone to its active form. In contrast to the SULTs, the major sites of expression are breast, ovary, prostate, testis and placenta. There are at least 17 of these enzymes, but one, steroid sulphatase (STS, also known as arylsulphatase C), is the primary enzyme involved in steroid desulphation. All sulphatases have a cysteine residue at the catalytic site that is converted to formylglycine by formylglycine generating enzyme, encoded by the *SUMF1* gene. The formylglycine residue is essential for binding the substrate and for hydrolysing the sulphate-ester bond. STS is predominantly, but not exclusively, located in the endoplasmic reticulum and is ubiquitous in expression with highest levels in the placenta. Activity may also be increased in some cancers and is thought to play a role in hormone-dependent tumour growth.

Both sulphotransferase and sulphatase play important roles in the fetoplacental unit. From 9 weeks of gestation, the placenta is the major source of maternal oestrogen. While this can be produced by de novo synthesis, it is insufficient and the bulk of the oestrogen is synthesised from maternal and fetal adrenal DHEAS and fetal liver 16αhydroxyDHEAS (16αOHDHEAS). The two conjugated steroids from the fetus are taken up by the placenta through specific transporters, OATP2B1 and OAT4, respectively. Maternal DHEAS is transported into the placenta by the sodium-dependant organic anion transporter (SOAT). STS in the syncytiotrophoblast (the epithelial covering of the placental villi) deconjugates DHEAS, and it is subsequently metabolised to placental oestrone and oestradiol by the action of 3β-hydroxysteroid dehydrogenase, aromatase and 17β-hydroxysteroid dehydrogenase. The 16αOHDHEAS that is almost all from the fetus is metabolised to oestriol, and the latter is therefore a measure of fetal well-being and placental function. As its synthesis is dependent on the desulphation of steroids in the placenta, measurement of maternal urinary oestriol can be used as a prenatal diagnostic test for STS deficiency (see Sect. 13.6). On the maternal side, oestriol is conjugated with glucuronic acid and excreted into the urine, oestrone is sulphated and oestradiol remains largely unconjugated. Unconjugated oestrogens diffusing from the placenta to the fetus are subsequently sulphated and therefore inactivated.

13.2 Presentation

There are no documented deficiency states of human steroid sulphotransferases perhaps reflecting the broad substrate specificity of these enzymes allowing compensation by other enzymes. Mouse models have shown that loss of the oestrogen sulphotransferase gene, *sult1e1*, causes placental thrombosis and mid-gestation embryo loss, but as yet no human disorders have been described. Deficiency of the essential sulphonation factor PAPSS2 has, however, been reported in a number of patients and presents with bone dysplasia and an increase in androgen activation through enhanced 5α-reductase activity. A polycystic ovary syndrome phenotype has also been described in affected females.

By contrast STS deficiency is relatively common with a prevalence of 1:1500–1:6000 males and leads to the skin disorder, X-linked ichthyosis, where the skin is typically covered in dark brown scales—the result of accumulation of sulphated sterols, mainly cholesterol sulphate, in the epidermis. More recently it has been shown that there is a spectrum of skin appearances ranging from dry skin and eczema through to light grey and dark brown scales. Additional features may be present, including autism and intellectual disability presumably reflecting the size of deletion on the X chromosome causing the disease and the number of other genes affected (see Sect. 13.3). The disorder appears to have no impact on pubertal development of the male although serum testosterone was found to be lower in post-pubertal patients with STS deficiency.

Fetal STS deficiency may also present in pregnancy with the finding of low maternal serum oestriol prompting investigations into fetal well-being.

13.3 Genetics

The chromosomal location of SULT genes of interest in steroid metabolism are given in Table 13.1. The *SULT2B1a* and *SULT2B1b* enzymes are encoded by *SULT2B1*. The genes differ at their 5′ termini and represent alternative transcripts. They are only 48% identical to *SULT2A1* and are 500 kb telomeric to that gene on the long arm of chromosome 19.

To date there are no documented mutations in these genes, but an association has been described with a single nucleotide polymorphism rs182420, an adenine to guanine change at the 3′ end of *SULT2A1*, that may contribute to lower serum DHEAS and act as a modifier of adrenal androgen production in polycystic ovary patients. It is not known whether this change affects a regulatory site that affects expression or is in linkage disequilibrium with an unknown functional variant elsewhere in the gene.

Mutations have been described in *PAPSS2*. This gene is located on the long arm of chromosome 10 at 10q23.2-q23.2. The mutations described include missense, nonsense and splice site changes. PAPSS2 activity has been shown to vary more than 18-fold between individuals, and extensive analysis has been performed to look for non-pathological variants that might contribute to such differences. Two non-synonymous variants have been described that do affect expression of the factor. One of these, p.Glu10Lys, when expressed in vitro shows reduced expression and decreased immunoreactive protein. The other change, p.Val291Met, had a decreased affinity for ATP but no reduction in immunoreactive protein.

The gene encoding STS, *STS*, is located on chromosome Xp22.3-Xpter. This gene escapes the X-inactivation process and thus deficiency is inherited as an autosomal recessive. The gene is 10 exons spanning 146 kb. The majority (80–90%) of mutations are caused by large deletions knocking out the whole gene and part of the flanking region. Additional features of the disease, e.g. autism and intellectual disability, may reflect the size of the deletion and the number of other genes affected. Some point mutations have been described that completely ablate enzyme activity.

13.4 Diagnosis

Unexplained hyperandrogenism from a suspected adrenal source may be the initial indicator for investigation of sulphotransferase or PAPSS2 deficiency, although the latter would probably also have additional evidence of bone dysplasia. DHEAS is typically low (<0.5 μmol/L) with an increased ratio of DHEA to DHEAS in the range 100:1 nmol/μmol, compared to a normal in the region of 4:1 nmol/μmol. In the UK DHEAS is usually routinely available as part of endocrinological investigations, but DHEA is only available in a few centres offering analysis by liquid chromatography-mass spectrometry, and therefore this ratio may not be available. However, failure of DHEAS to respond to a challenge with 100 mg DHEA is a strong indication of sulphotransferase or PAPSS2 deficiency.

For individuals with dermatological findings suggestive of steroid sulphatase deficiency, the most discriminating measurement is serum cholesterol sulphate that can be up to 36 times higher than that in controls. Serum androgens are similar in affected and controls, but urine DHEA metabolites tend to be higher in these patients. These metabolites reflect both conjugated and unconjugated DHEA, but in normal circumstances as 99% arises from DHEAS, they can be regarded as a reflection of DHEAS.

13.5 Case Study

A 32-year-old woman was found to have a serum oestriol of <0.3 medians of the mean on the second trimester antenatal screen. A fresh blood sample was taken and the low result confirmed. All other screen components of the quad test were normal for gestational age. She denied taking any corticosteroids that may lead to fetal adrenal suppression. An ultrasound scan of the fetus was performed to confirm fetal viability and to exclude anencephaly and in utero growth failure as a cause of the low oestriol, and an additional anomaly scan at 22 weeks did not show any dysmorphic features. A 24 h urine steroid profile from the mother confirmed significantly reduced oestriol output. Analysis of the sulphate fraction showed markedly increased 16αOHDHEA, androstenetriol and 16αOH pregnenolone thus excluding fetal adrenal failure or an adrenal biosynthetic defect. The results were consistent with placental sulphatase deficiency.

Her baby boy was born at term after a normal vaginal delivery. No further testing was performed at birth and he developed normally. At age 4 years, he presented to the dermatologist with grey scales covering his lower limbs consistent with ichthyosis.

13.6 Steroid Profile

Prenatal findings: A urine steroid profile is of most use for the prenatal diagnosis of STS deficiency where one is looking for a decrease in oestriol production in *maternal* urine indicating a failure of placental STS. Oestriol is approximately 10% of normal in the third trimester with values of 1.5 μg/24 h reported in STS deficiency compared with 12.5 μg/24 h in controls. To visualise the other abnormal metabolites, the urine sulphate fraction must be analysed separately to avoid overlap with some of the progesterone metabolites that are excreted as glucuronides. The sulphated metabolites are the fetal 3β-hydroxy-5-ene sulphates that are excreted unchanged and include 16αOHDHEA, androstenetriol and 16α-hydroxypregnenolone (Table 13.2). The mean output of these three steroids in the third trimester was 9210, 4710 and 2620 μg/24 h in placental sulphatase deficiency compared to 480, 330 and 80 μg/24 h in control pregnancies. Absence of these metabolites in conjunction with a decreased oestriol may indicate a possible adrenal biosynthetic or aromatase defect.

Table 13.2 Steroid metabolites in maternal urine used for assessment of placental sulphatase deficiency, retention times (methylene units, MU) of their MO-TMS derivatives and characteristic ions (see appendix for spectra)

Steroid	Trivial name	MU	Relevant ions
5-Androsten-3β,16α-diol-17-one	16αOHDHEA	27.38/27.42[a]	266, 446
5-Androsten-3β,16α,17β-triol	Androstenetriol	28.46	432, 329
Estra-1,3,5(10)-triene-3,16α,17β-triol	Oestriol	28.75	504, 386
5-Pregnen-3β,16α-diol-20-one	16α-Hydroxypregnenolone	29.38	474, 384

[a]Denotes the epimers

Postnatal findings in STS deficiency: The urine steroid profile from males with STS deficiency tends to show rather non-specific changes. For example, there is an increased ratio of 5α- to 5β-reduced glucocorticoid metabolites, i.e. 5α tetrahydrocortisol/tetrahydrocortisol. Values of approximately twice that seen in age matched controls have been reported in STS deficiency suggesting enhanced peripheral androgen synthesis. There was no overall difference in total androsterone + aetiocholanolone excretion in STS deficiency, but 24-h urinary DHEAS excretion was significantly elevated in pre- and post-pubertal subjects relative to controls.

Postnatal findings in PAPPS2 deficiency: Urine steroid profile from post-pubertal boys with PAPPS2 deficiency showed an excess of the 5α-metabolite, androsterone relative to aetiocholanolone, the 5α/5β ratio some two to three times that seen in controls. DHEA output, primarily reflecting DHEAS, was reduced. Following an oral DHEA challenge, the androsterone output was exaggerated reflecting an increase in active androgen production, but DHEAS output remained lower than that seen in controls.

13.7 Treatment

No specific treatments are available for these disorders.

Further Reading

Geyer J, Bakhaus K, Bernhardt R, et al. The role of sulfated steroid hormones in reproductive processes. J Steroid Biochem Mol Biol. 2017;172:207–21.

Reed LJ, Purohit A, Woo LWL, Newman SP, Potter BVL. Steroid sulfatase: molecular biology, regulation and inhibition. Endocr Rev. 2005;26:171–202.

14 Cholesterol Synthesis Defects

Francis Lam and Oliver Clifford-Mobley

14.1 Introduction

Steroid biosynthesis originates from cholesterol, and so it follows that disorders of cholesterol metabolism can also affect steroid hormone and bile acid production. Cholesterol is also an essential component of cell membranes, is part of myelin and is required for correct neurotransmitter function; hence deficiency can have far reaching consequences. The pathway of cholesterol synthesis is illustrated in Fig. 14.1. The first part of this multistep process, the isoprenoid pathway, converts acetate to farnesyl pyrophosphate. The second part, sterol synthesis, further metabolises farnesyl pyrophosphate to cholesterol. The enzyme 3-hydroxy-3-methylglutaryl coenzyme A (HMG CoA) reductase is the rate-limiting step in cholesterol biosynthesis.

The adrenal glands can synthesise cholesterol *de novo*, but the main source is from uptake of low-density lipoprotein (LDL) from plasma, a process mediated by the LDL receptor. Intracellular cholesterol concentrations are regulated by sterol response element-binding proteins (SREBPs) which are transcription factors that regulate genes involved in cholesterol homeostasis including those for the LDL receptor, which promotes the endocytosis of LDL cholesterol, and HMG CoA reductase. Esterified cholesterol is stored in lipid droplets and in the lysosomes. At least two enzymes have been shown to hydrolyse cholesteryl esters: hormone sensitive lyase and lysosomal acid lipase (LAL), mutations in the latter causing Wolman's and cholesteryl ester storage disease. Stimulation of steroidogenesis by adrenocorticotrophic hormone (ACTH) increases available cholesterol by promoting the

F. Lam (✉)
Manual Blood Sciences, Health Services Laboratories LLP, London, UK
e-mail: francis.lam@nhs.net

O. Clifford-Mobley
Department of Clinical Biochemistry, Bristol Royal Infirmary, University Hospitals Bristol, Bristol, UK

G. Rumsby, G. M. Woodward (eds.), *Disorders of Steroidogenesis*,
https://doi.org/10.1007/978-3-319-96364-8_14

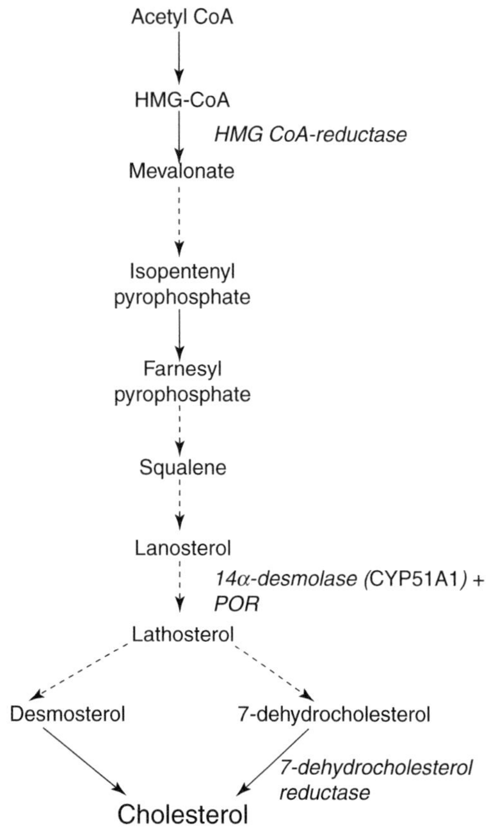

Fig. 14.1 Cholesterol synthesis from acetate. HMG CoA-reductase is the rate-limiting step. Reactions catalysed by 14α-desmolase (CYP51A1) and 7-dehydrocholesterol reductase are affected in cytochrome P450 oxidoreductase deficiency and Smith-Lemli-Opitz syndrome, respectively

uptake of LDL and hormone-sensitive lipase activity while decreasing the activity of the acyl-CoA/cholesterol acyltransferase enzyme. Cholesterol is then transferred to the mitochondria by a carrier-mediated process, one of which is the steroidogenic acute regulatory protein (see Chap. 8).

Wolman's and cholesteryl ester storage diseases are rare autosomal recessive disorders both caused by defects in LAL. Wolman's represents the more severe end of the disease spectrum with an estimated frequency of 1 in 350,000 and presents in the first year of life. Milder forms of disease, in which enzyme activity is at least 5–10% of normal, are thought to have a frequency of 1 in 50,000 and allow survival until adulthood. Loss of LAL activity confers an insufficient ability to hydrolyse stored lysosomal cholesteryl esters and triglycerides, and these accumulate in hepatocytes, adrenal, intestine and macrophage-monocyte cells. There is a compensatory upregulation of cholesterol synthesis and increased endocytosis by increasing the number of LDL receptors. There is also impairment of the membrane lipid transporter ATP-binding cassette transporter 1 (ABCA1) that impairs lipid efflux to HDL. The lack of sufficient free cholesterol substrate for the cytochrome P450 side chain cleavage enzyme results in inadequate steroidogenesis, and affected individuals can present with primary adrenal insufficiency as well as hepatosplenomegaly. Disease progression in

Wolman's disease leads to liver failure and adrenal insufficiency resulting in infant death, often within a few months. Less severe LAL deficiency may present in adulthood with hepatomegaly and may be misdiagnosed or even have a role in the more prevalent hepatic disorders such as non-alcoholic fatty liver disease. Continued hepatic damage can, however, progress to liver fibrosis, cirrhosis and liver failure.

Smith-Lemli-Opitz syndrome (SLOS) is caused by deficiency of 7-dehydrocholesterol reductase, encoded by *DHCR7*. It is inherited as an autosomal recessive trait and has an estimated incidence of approximately 1 in 60,000, making it the most common of the disorders of cholesterol biosynthesis. There is wide clinical variability of SLOS ranging from death *in utero* through to mild dysmorphic features. The inability to produce enough cholesterol for normal embryonic development can have a devastating impact on the fetus, and it is hypothesised that SLOS may be responsible for a large number of miscarriages. Cholesterol is required for correct functioning of the Sonic hedgehog (SHH) protein, which is an embryonic signalling complex. Inherited defects in SHH give rise to holoprosencephaly, which is a syndrome with dysmorphology similar to that of SLOS. The most common presenting defect in males with SLOS is genital abnormality (91%) ranging from hypospadias to ambiguous genitalia along with other dysmorphic features including syndactyly of second and third toes (81%), microcephaly (80%), anteverted nares (69%), low-set ears (47%) and small jaw (micrognathia) (67%). Congenital heart defects and learning difficulties are also common.

Intuitively SLOS might be expected to cause deficiency of all the steroid hormones due to reduced substrate (cholesterol) availability. Primary adrenal insufficiency can indeed be a feature of SLOS but it is rare and only seen in the more severe cases. Under-virilisation of 46, XY individuals with SLOS can by this same logic be attributed to reduced sex steroid biosynthesis.

The severity of SLOS correlates with serum cholesterol levels (i.e. as a surrogate marker for residual endogenous synthesis), and furthermore treatment with cholesterol supplementation can improve symptoms for affected patients, sometimes dramatically. This provides evidence that the pathogenesis of SLOS is directly related to the cholesterol deficiency.

Cytochrome P450 oxidoreductase (POR) is a membrane-bound flavoprotein that receives electrons from NADPH and transfers them to a number of cytochrome P450 enzymes. The investigation of patients with Antley-Bixler syndrome (ABS), a rare disorder characterised by craniosynostosis, midface hypoplasia and distinct facial anomalies as well as genital ambiguity, required an overarching explanation for the findings of impaired steroidogenesis seen in this disorder. Multiple enzymes are affected including lanosterol 14α-demethylase (CYP51A1), required for cholesterol synthesis, and 21- and 17α-hydroxylases needed for cortisol and androgen biosynthesis, respectively. POR is a common cofactor for these enzymes, and mutations in *POR* subsequently confirmed its role in at least some cases of ABS. It is also possible to have ABS without adrenal insufficiency. In these cases, loss of function variants in the fibroblast growth factor receptor 2 (FGFR2) are the underlying cause. POR deficiency is inherited as an autosomal recessive trait and is extremely rare with only about 100 cases known worldwide.

Impaired androgen synthesis in POR deficiency means that 46, XY patients can be born with ambiguous genitalia and are under-virilised. It is therefore interesting to observe that 46, XX patients can be virilised, suggesting exposure to excess androgens *in utero*. In some cases, the mothers of an affected fetus have reported virilisation that reverses following delivery. It is suggested that attenuated aromatase activity (another enzyme that uses POR as a cofactor) may account for some of the virilising effects but against this is the absence of metabolites characteristic of aromatase deficiency in maternal urine: 16α-hydroxyandrosterone and 16α-hydroxyaetiocholanolone. Androgens have also been postulated to arise from an alternative steroid pathway in which androsterone and dihydrotestosterone are formed from 17-hydroxyprogesterone (see Chap. 4). After birth no further virilisation occurs, and there is oestrogen deficiency causing hypergonadotropic hypogonadism. Ovarian cysts may be present in the adult female with POR deficiency, mimicking PCOS.

14.2 Presentation

Wolman's and cholesteryl ester storage disease present with hepatomegaly and splenomegaly, in the former case with fatal consequences within the first year of life. Milder deficiencies may not present until adulthood with symptoms related to liver cirrhosis with confirmation of excess lipid storage in a liver biopsy.

SLOS typically presents with genital ambiguity along with other characteristic dysmorphic features as previously described. Feeding difficulties are common. The disorder may also be suspected *in utero* from the finding of decreased maternal serum oestriol and abnormal ultrasound findings including increased nuchal translucency, ambiguous genitalia and polydactyly.

Deficiency of POR can lead to a range of clinical features, depending on the degree of loss of enzyme activity. There is an isolated adrenal phenotype, a polycystic ovarian syndrome (PCOS)-like phenotype and also a dysmorphic phenotype similar to ABS, the latter occurring in four-fifths of cases, but in contrast to ABS caused by FGFR2 mutations, genital ambiguity is also seen as an additional feature.

Adrenal only POR deficiency is a very rare subtype of CAH, which has been reported in only a handful of cases. Affected individuals present with the biochemical features that might be expected from combined 21-hydroxylase and 17α-hydroxylase deficiency CAH, i.e. defective synthesis of both glucocorticoids and sex hormones. The deficiency of glucocorticoids can make the patient vulnerable to an adrenal crisis and requires treatment with exogenous steroids. The loss of normal negative feedback in the hypothalamic-pituitary-adrenal axis leads to increased synthesis of adrenocorticotrophic hormone (ACTH) which drives the adrenal hyperplasia. In common with 21-hydroxylase deficiency, a 'partial block' can be seen with the patient able to synthesise some endogenous cortisol. However, this is insufficient for times of acute stress and comes at the expense of the ACTH excess. Salt loss due to reduced mineralocorticoids is not normally part of the clinical spectrum, and this may be due to increased deoxycorticosterone production secondary to the 17-hydroxylase deficiency.

14.3 Genetics

The *LIPA* gene encoding LAL is located on chromosome 10q23.31 and a range of mutations have been described. The most common variant is c.894G>A that occurs in the last nucleotide of exon 8 and causes missplicing of the mRNA. Approximately 3–5% of the transcripts are correctly spliced and therefore some residual activity is maintained. Another mutation, p.Gly87Val has been described in both Wolman's and cholesteryl ester storage disease and appears to be a founder variant in people of Iranian-Jewish ancestry.

DHCR7 encoding 7-dehydrocholesterol reductase is located on chromosome 11q13.4. More than 150 pathogenic variants have been described. Unsurprisingly those mutations that cause complete loss of enzyme activity are associated with the most severe phenotype of SLOS. The most common pathological variant occurring in 28% of disease alleles is c.832-1G>C (IVS8-1G>C), a splice site acceptor mutation that causes incorrect splicing and premature stop codon. The majority of other variants are missense changes.

The *POR* gene on chromosome 7q11.23 is composed of 15 exons and encodes a protein of 681 amino acids with four functional domains. A variety of mutations have been described. One common benign variant, p.Ala503Val, occurring at a frequency of 27% in the normal population, shows a modest but significant decrease in the activity of 17α-hydroxylase and may contribute to interindividual differences in metabolism. The variant did not, however, influence the activity of 21-hydroxylase. The missense change, p.Ala287Pro accounts for approximately 40% of mutations in individuals of European origin and leads to a fall in 17α-hydroxylase to 20–40% of wild-type but only a 30% reduction in 21-hydroxylase activity. The p.Arg457His variant, which accounts for around 60% pathogenic variants in Japan, disrupts both 17α- and 21-hydroxylase activities to a similar degree.

14.4 Diagnosis

Patients with Wolman's disease typically have elevated serum total cholesterol, LDL-cholesterol, triglycerides and transaminases, but HDL-cholesterol is usually low. Confirmation of the disease requires measurement of LAL activity in either leucocytes or dried blood spot samples. In the latter, total lipase activity is first measured followed by reanalysis in the presence of a lysosomal acid lipase inhibitor. The difference between the two measurements is attributed to LAL.

Initial investigations in a patient with suspected SLOS includes measurement of serum cholesterol that is typically low although about 10% of cases will have levels within the reference range, a situation that may reflect cross reaction of 7-dehydrocholesterol in the serum cholesterol assay. The definitive diagnosis is by measurement of 7-dehydrocholesterol which is elevated, typically 50-fold above normal although lower values have been shown. A urine steroid profile can also be helpful (see Sect. 14.6).

Depending on the presentation, the differential diagnosis of POR deficiency may include other forms of CAH as well as Antley-Bixler syndrome and other disorders with similar dysmorphology. In cases where adrenal impairment is suspected, serum cortisol and ACTH measurements are required. 17-Hydroxyprogesterone is often above the reference range with some reports of values >100 nmol/L suggestive of

21-hydroxylase deficiency although it is not clear what methodology was used for the measurement in these reports. If taken in the newborn period, these results may reflect interference from other steroids. Where there is residual POR activity, stimulation of the hypothalamic-pituitary-adrenal axis with a short Synacthen test may be required to make the diagnosis of adrenal insufficiency. A urine steroid profile is an extremely useful test for assessment of all forms of CAH. As detailed below in Sect. 14.6, a mixed picture of 21- and 17α-hydroxylase deficiencies is evident in POR deficiency. Confirmation by genetic testing allows future prenatal diagnosis.

14.5 Case Study

A full-term newborn was noted to have micrognathia and syndactyly with additional dysmorphology. SLOS was suspected. Serum cholesterol was low (1.2 mmol/L, reference range for newborns 1.7 ± 0.27) and serum 7-dehydrocholesterol elevated at 800 μmol/L (reference range <2). A urine was taken for urine steroid profile and showed the characteristic metabolites of 7-dehydrocholesterol and 8-dehydrocholesterol (see Fig. 14.2).

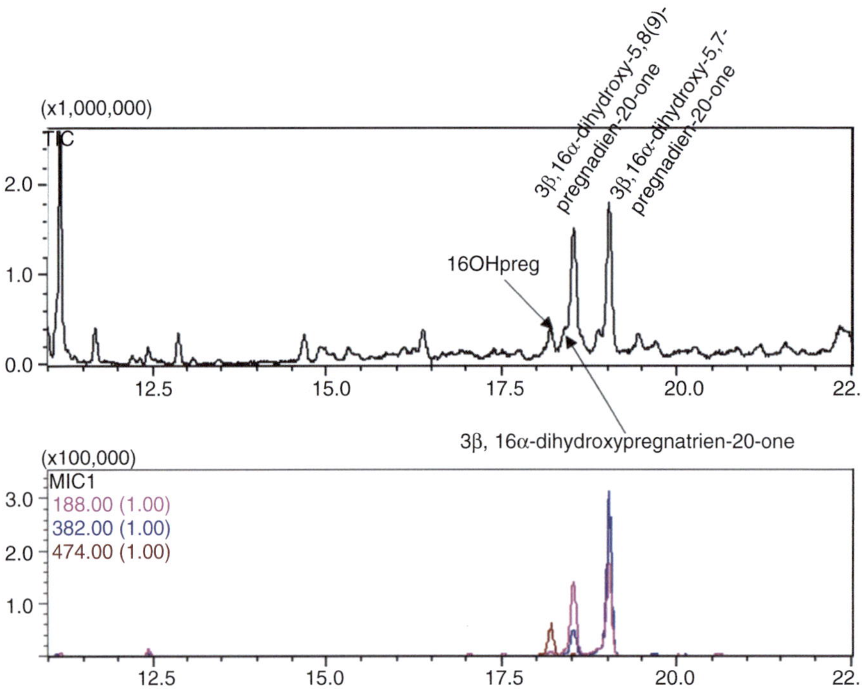

Fig. 14.2 Urine steroid sulphate fraction from neonate with SLOS. (**a**) Total ion count showing cluster of SLOS-related metabolites eluting just after 16α OH pregnenolone (16αOHPe). (**b**) Selective ion monitoring for m/z 382 seen in 3β,16α-dihydroxy-5,8(9)-pregnadien-20-one and 3β,16α-dihydroxy-5,7-pregnadien-20-one. 16αOHPe (m/z 474) is included as a reference. 3β,16α-Dihydroxypregnatrien-20-one is a shoulder on the side of 3β,16α-dihydroxy-5,8(9)-pregnadien-20-one

14.6 Steroid Profile

LAL deficiency has no specific steroid profile associated with it other than a decreased output of all adrenal steroids.

The steroid sulphate fraction of urine from SLOS patients is characterised by metabolites of 7- and 8-dehydrocholesterol, the latter possibly arising from the action of a Δ^7–Δ^8 isomerase (Table 14.1). The metabolites are the unsaturated homologues of the dominant, usually 16α-hydroxylated, neonatal steroids, and are evidence that the dehydrocholesterols are also substrates for the cholesterol 20-22 lyase enzyme. In the SLOS neonate, there is a marked decrease in 3β-hydroxy-5-ene steroids that are the primary output from the fetal adrenal with 16α-hydroxypregnenolone (16αOHPe) and 16α-hydroxydehydroepiandrosterone (16αOHDHEA) being approximately 10% of normal. In addition, a number of unsaturated steroids are found of which three dehydro homologues of 16α-hydroxypregnenolone particularly stand out in the profile and elute immediately after 16αOHPe. The first of these, 3β,16α-dihydroxypregnatrien-20-one, elutes just after 16αOHPe (Fig. 14.2). The second and third metabolites, 3β,16α-dihydroxy-5,8(9)-pregnadien-20-one and 3β,16α-dihydroxy-5,7-pregnadien-20-one (Fig. 14.2), have the same ions but differ in their abundance. In both cases the molecular ion is *m/z* 503 with the major ion at 382 (M-90-31).

In utero diagnosis of SLOS: Reduced maternal serum oestriol and an abnormal scan may point to SLOS *in utero*. Some of the 7- and 8-dehydro metabolites are present in maternal urine including Δ^7 homologues of pregnanetriol and 7-dehydrooestriol that can be detected by selective ion monitoring (Table 14.1). In SLOS, dehydropregnanetriol/pregnanetriol ratios of 0.037–1.02 were found compared to <0.01 in unaffected pregnancies between 14 and 22 weeks gestation. Similarly 7-dehydro-oestriol/oestriol ratios of 0.073–1.42 were found in SLOS (normal <0.01). A USP of maternal urine can therefore be used for non-invasive prenatal diagnosis.

Table 14.1 Steroid metabolites excreted in SLOS and in maternal urine in pregnancies affected by SLOS, retention times (methylene units, MU) of their MO-TMS derivatives and characteristic ions (see appendix for spectra)

Steroid	Trivial name	MU	Characteristic ions
5-Androsten-3β,16α-diol-17-one	16α OHDHEA	27.38/27.42	266, 446
5-Pregnen-3β,16α-diol-20-one	16α OH pregnenolone	29.38	474, 384
3β,16α-Dihydroxypregnatrien-20-one		29.61	380, 290
3β,16α-Dihydroxy-5,8(9)-pregnadien-20-one		29.68	382
3β,16α-Dihydroxy-5,7-pregnadien-20-one		30.00	382
Maternal urine			
5β-Pregnane-3α,17α,20α-triol	Pregnanetriol	28.00	255, 435
5β-Pregn-7-ene-3α,17α,20α-triol	Dehydropregnanetriol	28.00	343, 253
1,3,5-Oestratriene-3β,17β-diol	Oestriol	28.75	504, 386
1,3,5(10),7-Oestratetraene-3,16α,17β-triol	7-Dehydrooestriol	28.75	502, 412, 397, 322

Table 14.2 Steroid metabolites of use for the diagnosis of POR deficiency, retention times (methylene units, MU) of their MO-TMS derivatives and characteristic ions (see appendix for spectra)

Steroid	Trivial name	MU	Characteristic ions
Pregna-5,20-dien-3β-ol	Pregnadienol artefact		357, 372
5-Androsten-3β,16α-diol-17-one	16αOHDHEA	27.38/27.42	446, 266
3α,17α-Dihydroxy-5β-pregnan-20-one	17α-OH pregnanolone	27.02	476, 188
5β-Pregnane-3α,20α-diol	Pregnanediol	27.72	117, 269
5-Pregnene-3β,20α-diol	Pregnenediol	28.16	117, 372
3α,17α,20α-Trihydroxy-5β-pregnan-11-one	11-Oxopregnanetriol	29.10	449, 359
3α,16α-Dihydroxy-5-pregnen-20-one	16αOH pregnenolone	29.38	474, 384
5-Pregnene-3β,17α,20α-triol	Δ5-Pregnenetriol	29.46	253, 433
3α,17α,21-Trihydroxy-5β-pregnan-11,20-dione	THE	29.65	578, 488
3α,21-Dihydroxy-5β-pregnan-11,20-dione	THA	29.77	188, 400
3α,11β,21-Trihydroxy-5β-pregnan-20-one	THB	30.00	188, 564
3α,11β,21-Trihydroxy-5α-pregnan-20-one	5αTHB	30.16	188, 474
Maternal urine			
5α-Pregn-17(20)-en-3β-ol	Epiallopregnenol	Before androsterone	
5α-Pregnane-3β,20α-diol	Epiallopregnanediol		
5β-Pregnane-3α,20α-diol	Pregnanediol	27.72	117, 269

In POR deficiency some cortisol metabolites are usually present, frequently at the low end of normal, presumably reflecting residual activity of the cytosolic 21- and 17α-hydroxylase P450 enzymes that utilise POR as an electron carrier. A list of relevant metabolites is given in Table 14.2.

In the neonatal sulphate fraction, 16αOHPe is disproportionately higher than 16αOHDHEA consistent with impaired 17α-hydroxylase activity. The characteristic urine biomarkers for POR deficiency are elevated excretion of pregnenediol and pregnanediol, the major urinary metabolites of pregnenolone and progesterone, respectively (Fig. 14.3). In addition, markers of 21-hydroxylase deficiency (pregnanetriol, 17α-hydroxypregnanolone and 11-oxopregnanetriol) may also be present. The corticosterone metabolite, α-tetrahydrocorticosterone (αTHB), also tends to be elevated when cortisol metabolites are present suggesting that 21-hydroxylase activity is less susceptible to POR deficiency than 17α-hydroxylase. Pregnadienol, an artefact formed from pregnenediol disulphate is present in the early part of the spectrum, particularly in cases with the ABS phenotype perhaps reflecting the severity of the defect.

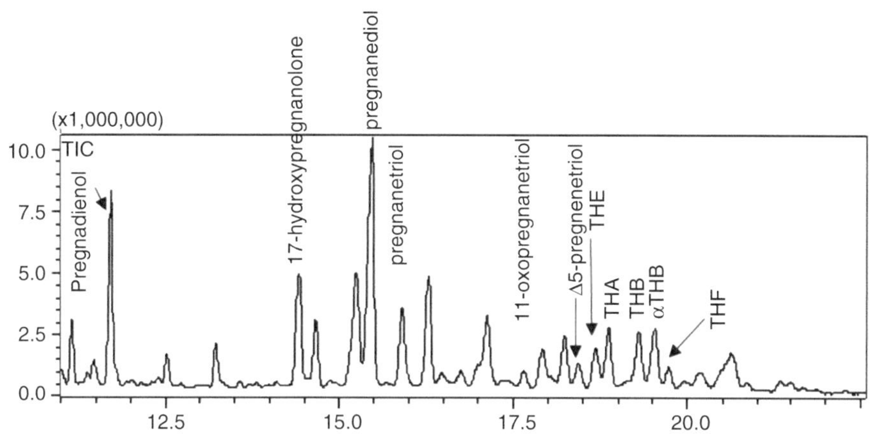

Fig. 14.3 Total ion current chromatogram of urine steroids from patient with POR deficiency. Markers of both 21-hydroxylase and 17α-hydroxylase deficiency are present along with some cortisol metabolites. The pregnadienol metabolite at the front of the spectrum is characteristic of the disorder

Various ratios of metabolites have been suggested to act as diagnostic indicators of POR deficiency. For one of these, pregnanediol/(THE + THF + 5αTHF), ratios of 0.35–0.80 have been described in POR patients, whereas normals are approximately 0.1. In addition, a low excretion of 11β-hydroxyandrosterone has also been described in this disorder.

It has been reported that prenatal diagnosis is possible using a maternal USP, with the steroid metabolite epiallopregnanediol (5α-pregnane-3β,20α-diol) being specifically elevated. This steroid is an abnormal metabolite of 5-pregnene-3β,20α-diol, the principal metabolite of fetal pregnenolone and reflects the metabolic block present in the feto-placental unit. As a consequence of this block maternal oestriol concentrations are low. The epiallopregnanediol disulphate forms an artefact, epiallopregnenol, following hydrolysis and derivatisation that elutes in a similar position to androsterone at the start of the chromatogram.

14.7 Treatment

A human enzyme replacement for LAL deficiency, sebelipase, is in clinical trials and has shown some benefit on atherogenic markers, in particular with reduction of LDL-cholesterol. Other lipid-lowering measures have been tried with limited success. Liver transplantation has not been shown to halt disease progression.

Some cases of SLOS have been shown to respond to cholesterol replacement with improvements in weight gain, but this has no benefit to developmental progress. The use of statins, to prevent *de novo* cholesterol synthesis to minimise the accumulation of precursors, in conjunction with cholesterol replacement also failed to show any benefit on growth or behaviour of patients.

Patients with POR deficiency may require replacement with glucocorticoids particularly in periods of acute stress or illness, but doses given can be lower than for 21-hydroxylase deficiency as they are not required to also suppress adrenal androgen excess.

Further Reading

More About the POR Enzyme and Effect of Mutations

Huang N, Agrawal V, Giacomini KM, Miller WL. Genetics of P450 oxidoreductase: sequence variation in 842 individuals of four ethnicities and activities of 15 missense mutations. Proc Natl Acad Sci U S A. 2008;105:1733–8.

Miller WL, Huang N, Agrawal V, Giacomini KM. Genetic variation in human P450 oxidoreductase. Mol Cell Endocrinol. 2009;300:180–4.

Prenatal Metabolites Found in POR

Shackleton C, Marcos J, Arlt W, Hauffa BP. Prenatal diagnosis of P450 oxidoreductase deficiency (ORD): a disorder causing low pregnancy estriol, maternal and fetal virilization, and the Antley–Bixler syndrome phenotype. Am J Med Genet A. 2004;129A:105–12.

SLOS

Prenatal Metabolites

Shackleton CH, Roitman E, Kratz LE, Kelley RI. Equine type estrogens produced by a pregnant woman carrying a Smith–Lemli–Opitz syndrome fetus. J Clin Endocrinol Metab. 1999;84:1157–9.

Shackleton CH, Roitman E, Kratz LE, Kelley RI. Midgestational maternal urine steroid markers of fetal Smith–Lemli–Opitz (SLO) syndrome (7-dehydrocholesterol 7-reductase deficiency). Steroids. 1999;64:446–52.

Steroid-Producing Tumours 15

Gill Rumsby

15.1 Introduction

Excess hormone production by the adrenal glands can occur as a result of adrenal hyperplasia secondary to excess adrenocorticotrophic hormone (ACTH) exposure, as, for example, in Cushing's disease or ectopic ACTH secretion. It can also arise from an autonomously producing mass in the adrenal gland itself, either an adenoma or carcinoma, or as a result of metastases to the adrenal gland. With the advent of computerised tomography (CT) and magnetic resonance imaging (MRI), there has been an increase in the incidental finding of masses >1 cm in size in the adrenal gland on abdominal imaging for some completely unrelated reason. These so-called incidentalomas are estimated to be present in up to 3% of adults in middle age rising to as high as 10% at age 70 years. The vast majority of these are non-functional and benign, but around 15% may autonomously produce hormone(s) and may be benign or malignant – a mixture of adenoma 41%, metastases 19%, adrenocortical carcinoma 10%, myelolipoma 9% and phaeochromocytoma 8%. Urine steroid profiles are useful for evaluating the functionality and may aid classification of such tumours.

Acquired adrenal hyperplasia is often the result of chronic ACTH exposure as seen in Cushing's disease and ectopic ACTH secretion. In more than 60% of cases, the adrenals appear symmetrically enlarged under CT, and this reflects the sustained tropic and mitogenic stimulus of ACTH or other peptides produced by the proopiomelanocortin (POMC) protein. Cushing's disease can also lead to unilateral adrenal adenomas as can poorly controlled congenital adrenal hyperplasia. ACTH-independent disease tends to present with unilateral rather than bilateral adrenal tumours although this situation is influenced by the underlying genetic change (see Sect. 15.3). Adrenal adenomas are benign, but, if functional, they may

G. Rumsby
Department of Clinical Biochemistry, University College London Hospitals, London, UK
e-mail: gill.rumsby@nhs.net

G. Rumsby, G. M. Woodward (eds.), *Disorders of Steroidogenesis*,
https://doi.org/10.1007/978-3-319-96364-8_15

still cause considerable morbidity through their metabolic effects. By contrast adrenal carcinomas are malignant, and, in general, these have a poor prognosis and are difficult to treat. Hypercortisolism is the presenting feature in 50–80% of adrenal neoplasms and hyperandrogenism in 40–60% with symptoms such as rapid-onset male-pattern baldness, hirsutism, virilisation and menstrual irregularities.

Adrenal carcinomas are rare with an incidence of 1 in 1.7 million. The prevalence of 2% in the general population increases to 7% in 70 year olds. The tumour tissue is dedifferentiated and often produces excess steroid precursors that may not be detected by serum hormone measurements but are evident on a urine steroid profile.

Endocrinologically active gonadal tumours are rare. Testicular tumours that have a syncytiotrophoblast cell component, including some seminomas and mixed germ cell tumours, produce excess human chorionic gonadotrophin (hCG). This hormone can stimulate testosterone and oestradiol synthesis. In addition, Leydig cell tumours, the most common of the non-germ cell testicular tumours, tend to produce excess oestradiol as a result of aromatase action on testosterone. Testicular adrenal rest tumours (TARTs) arise in patients with congenital adrenal hyperplasia and reflect the effects of excess stimulation by ACTH on cells in the testicular hilum. These cells are thought to arise from the common adrenal-gonadal primordium and migrate to the testis or may reflect a totipotent embryonic cell with both adrenal and testicular features. These cells maintain adrenocortical characteristics including the presence of ACTH receptors. TARTs are usually bilateral and this feature helps to differentiate them from Leydig cell tumours. In some cases, the presence of TART as a cause of testicular enlargement has led to a late diagnosis of congenital adrenal hyperplasia. TART can lead to hypogonadism as the output of steroids can suppress gonadotrophin production.

Rapid-onset virilisation in a female may be an indicator of an ovarian tumour of sex cord/stromal origin. Although these are usually benign, the degree of virilisation can be marked leading to menstrual irregularities, excessive hair growth and male-pattern baldness. Investigation needs to exclude potential adrenal causes of virilisation. In the postmenopausal female, hyperandrogenism may reflect either ovarian hyperthecosis or a virilising tumour. While most cases of trophoblastic disease do not cause a change in steroid excretion over that seen in non-pregnant conditions, cases complicated by theca lutein cysts can show an increase in androgen metabolites, pregnanediol and pregnanetriol and 17-hydroxypregnanolone in a pattern similar, but not identical, to 21-hydroxylase deficiency.

The evaluation of an adrenal or gonadal mass includes imaging, biochemical testing and histological assessment.

Imaging: CT scanning can determine the size and shape of the mass and also the density relative to water in terms of Hounsfield units (HU). On a non-enhanced scan, HU give an indication as to the lipid content of the mass. If $\leq$10 HU, it suggests a greater lipid content and is more in keeping with an adenoma rather than carcinoma or metastases. However, at least 30% of adenomas may be misclassified on density alone, and imaging does not give any information regarding functionality. In addition, a small percentage of malignant masses will be misclassified. Adenomas are typically of a smooth shape, are small (<4 cm) with encapsulated borders and have a homogeneous appearance on scanning. By contrast, carcinomas tend to be larger (greater than 4–5 cm), are of irregular shape, appear heterogeneous and may show signs of calcification. Their density is typically >18 HU although there may be some overlap with benign masses. In the case of masses greater than 10 HU, CT with intravenous contrast material is used and the washout of contrast material determined. Adenomas typically demonstrate more than 50% washout of contrast material at 10 min post administration, while metastases tend to be much lower.

Magnetic resonance imaging (MRI) is also used. Adenomas show a low signal on a T2-weighted image, whereas phaeochromocytomas have a brighter signal. Chemical shift MRI – a form of lipid-sensitive imaging – has also been used to differentiate between benign and malignant tissue.

Additional imaging using [^{18}F] fluorodeoxyglucose positron emission tomography is a highly sensitive and specific means of identifying metastatic disease in the adrenal gland detecting metabolically active tissue. The fluorodeoxyglucose is taken into cells in the same way as glucose and is phosphorylated by hexokinase but cannot be further metabolised, instead remaining trapped in the cell.

Histology: Malignancy can be assessed by analysis of the neoplasm, either by needle biopsy or more usually, following removal of the mass. The modified Weiss system (Table 15.1) is used by histologists for separating benign from malignant adrenocortical neoplasms.

Biochemical assessment: By definition, incidentalomas may well be asymptomatic, and investigation will need to include a variety of hormone measurements. Patients who present with symptoms possibly relating to the mass, e.g. hypertension, can be dealt with using a more focussed approach to exclude hyperaldosteronism, phaeochromocytoma and Cushing's syndrome. In the case of adrenal carcinoma, around 60–70% of tumours will overproduce hormones, but often these are steroid precursors as a result of dedifferentiation of the tumour often with loss of 3β-hydroxysteroid dehydrogenase, 11-hydroxylase and sulphotransferase activities. These precursors, including dehydroepiandrosterone (DHEA) and 11-deoxycortisol, will be evident in a urine steroid profile.

Table 15.1 Modified Weiss system for separating benign and malignant neoplasms

Scoring system: 2 × mitotic rate + 2 × cytoplasm + abnormal mitoses + necrosis + capsular invasion. A score of 3 or greater correlates with subsequent malignant behaviour
Mitotic rate – >5 per 50 high power fields
Cytoplasm (clear cells comprising 25% or less of the tumour)
Abnormal mitoses
Necrosis
Capsular invasion

15.2 Presentation

Presentation will typically reflect the type of steroid produced in excess. Hypercortisolism, for example, can lead to a Cushingoid habitus with truncal obesity, proximal muscle wasting, hypertension and diabetic symptoms. Those tumours that give rise to excess androgens may present with hirsutism, male-pattern baldness and menstrual irregularities in females, carcinomas typically having a rapid onset of virilisation. Gonadal tumours are generally less endocrinologically active and may actually present with symptoms of hypogonadism.

15.3 Genetics

Exome and next-generation sequencing have been used to study the genetic make-up of adrenal adenomas and carcinomas, and, in a number of cases, mutations have been found in proteins involved in the cAMP signalling cascade. This cascade starts with the binding of ACTH to the G-protein-coupled receptor and subsequent activation of adenyl cyclase, synthesis of cyclic AMP (cAMP) and interaction of this with the regulatory unit of protein kinase A (PKA) with subsequent release of the PKA catalytic subunit and phosphorylation of downstream targets including β-catenin.

In one-third of cortisol-producing adenomas, hyperplasia was caused by activating mutations in the *PRKACA* gene encoding the catalytic subunit of the cAMP-dependent PKA protein and downstream systems leading to constitutive PKA activity. Bilateral macronodular hyperplasia has been found associated with somatic mutations in *GNAS1* that lead to constitutive activation of the alpha subunit of the stimulatory G-protein that activates adenylate cyclase.

In adrenal adenomas there are three main pathways affected by mutations: (1) the cAMP/protein kinase A pathway, (2) Wnt/β catechin pathway and (3) Ca^{2+}-dependent signalling. One particular missense mutation in *PRKACA*, p.Leu206Arg, leads to disruption of the interaction between the regulatory subunit and the catalytic cleft of PKA, the end result being constitutive activation of PKA and cell proliferation. This mutation was found in the heterozygous state in 37% of cases with overt Cushing's syndrome. When present in the tumour alone, i.e. a somatic mutation, the disease was unilateral, but when present in the germ line, the tumours tended to be bilateral. Germ line mutations have also been described where duplication of part of chromosome 19 encompassing *PRKACA* occurs, presumably also leading to gain of function. Somatic activating mutations in *CTNNB1*, encoding β-catenin, and in *GNAS1* have also been described in some cortisol-secreting and non-functional adenomas. It is not yet clear why these activating mutations do not always lead to excess hormone secretion.

Adrenocortical carcinomas have mutations in a number of different genes affecting three major pathways, β-catechin pathway, P53/Rb signalling and chromatin remodelling, and include the genes *CTNNB1*, *TP53*, *CDKN2A*, *RB1*, *MEN1*, *ZNRF3*, *DAXX*, *TERT* and *MED12*. The most frequently altered gene was *ZNRF3*, encoding a cell surface E3 ubiquitin ligase 6 that acts as a negative feedback on β-catechin. Tumours with mutations in this gene exhibited activation of the β-catechin pathway.

In adults around 10% of adrenal carcinomas are associated with familial cancer predisposition syndromes including Li-Fraumeni (TP53 mutations), Lynch syndrome (mismatch repair genes), multiple endocrine neoplasia type 1 (*MENIN*), Beckwith-Wiedemann and familial adenomatous polyposis. Mutations in these genes are much more common in paediatric tumours where more than 70% contain mutations in the tumour suppressor, *TP53*.

Activating mutations in *GNAS* have also been demonstrated in some ovarian and testicular stromal luteal cell tumours.

15.4 Diagnosis

The presentation of an adrenal or gonadal mass may be an incidental finding on imaging or may be symptomatic of hormone excess. Diagnosis therefore needs to be performed in a logical manner.

Biochemical assessment should be carried out to evaluate the patient for a functional mass and will include tests to look for hyperaldosteronism, phaeochromocytoma and Cushing's syndrome in the first instance. Other symptoms, such as hirsutism, may suggest an androgen-secreting tumour of the adrenal or gonads. An algorithm for the investigation of an incidental adrenal mass is given in Fig. 15.1.

If the patient is hypertensive, the finding of a suppressed renin with aldosterone >300 pmol/L is highly suggestive of hyperaldosteronism (Conn's syndrome) assuming not on any interfering medication. The calcium channel blockers and alpha-blockers appear to have least effects on renin and aldosterone and, if possible, should be used for treatment of hypertension while investigations are carried out. Confirmation of autonomous aldosterone excess can be made by means of a saline

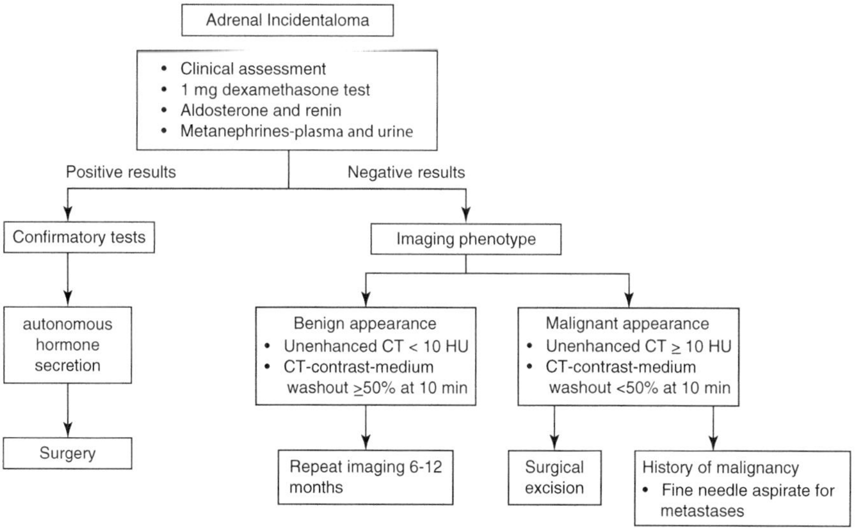

Fig. 15.1 Algorithm for the investigation of an adrenal incidentaloma

suppression test. It may be necessary to carry out adrenal vein sampling to determine whether the excess aldosterone is the result of a unilateral adenoma or bilateral adrenal hyperplasia. This investigation can be quite difficult to perform as cannulation of the adrenal veins requires significant expertise. The ratio of aldosterone to cortisol in the right and left adrenal veins is compared to that in the peripheral sample.

Hypertension (sustained or episodic) may also be an indicator of phaeochromocytoma particularly if accompanied by pallor and tremor. These tumours account for 5–8% of incidentalomas and may be asymptomatic at the time of finding. Measurement of plasma and/or urine metanephrines is essential for the diagnosis of phaeochromocytoma. Confirmatory testing usually requires metaiodobenzylguanidine (MIBG) scintigraphy.

Measurement of serum cortisol following 1 mg dexamethasone overnight is the initial test to exclude cortisol excess. If no suppression, then further tests including urine free cortisol on at least two occasions or salivary cortisol should be performed to investigate for Cushing's syndrome (see Chap. 16).

If the patient has symptoms such as hirsutism or oligomenorrhoea, it is sensible to measure other steroid hormones including testosterone and androstenedione along with a urine steroid profile to exclude undiagnosed congenital adrenal hyperplasia or androgen-secreting tumours. Exogenous sources of raised testosterone should be excluded including possible exposure to a partner's transdermal testosterone gel. Postmenopausal virilisation may be due to ovarian hyperthecosis or a virilising ovarian tumour. Reduction of testosterone by 50% on treatment with gonadotropin analogue would suggest an ovarian cause. If no suppression, then an adrenal source should be considered. The measurement of DHEAS can be helpful as if elevated it may suggest an adrenal tumour, but this has poor sensitivity. A urine steroid profile should also be performed in any case where an adrenal carcinoma is suspected.

15.5 Case Study

A 51-year-old hypertensive male (blood pressure 147/93 mmHg) was referred to the endocrine consultants following the discovery of a 14.7 cm adrenal incidentaloma that was of mixed density and 47 HU. Initial suspicion was of a phaeochromocytoma as, in addition to the hypertension, he had episodes of sweating, but no headaches or bowel disturbances were documented. He was on treatment with amlodipine and doxazosin. There was no family history of endocrine tumours. An ECG was normal and an echocardiogram showed no ventricular hypertrophy.

On investigation, plasma metanephrines showed a slightly elevated normetanephrine of 1472 pmol/L (<1180), but this normalised on repeat testing after resting for 30 min prior to collection of blood sample. An MIBG scan was negative. These results made a diagnosis of phaeochromocytoma unlikely.

Following 1 mg dexamethasone overnight, serum cortisol was 344 nmol/L, i.e. it had failed to suppress. A urine steroid profile showed output of cortisol metabolites approximately ten times normal and a significant output of intermediates including tetrahydro-11-deoxycortisol (THS), pregnenetriol (5-pregnene-3β,17α,20α-triol) and DHEA – all suggestive of adrenal carcinoma.

The tumour was removed and histology was consistent with an adrenocortical carcinoma. The tumour had a Weiss score of 7 (>3 consistent with malignant behaviour). The Ki-67 score, an indicator of cellular proliferation, was up to 10% (normal <0.2).

15.6 Steroid Profile

As mentioned above, adrenal carcinomas often show dedifferentiation and selectively lose 3β-hydroxysteroid dehydrogenase and 11-hydroxylase activities so the pattern tends to be dominated by Δ5 steroids.

Several studies have evaluated the role of steroid profiles in discriminating between adenomas and carcinomas. It has been recognised for some years that excess excretion of the 11-deoxycortisol metabolite, tetrahydro-11-deoxycortisol (THS), is an indicator of malignancy and this has been confirmed by computational analysis in larger groups of patients where THS, pregnenetriol (Δ5P3, 5-pregnene-3β,17α,20α-triol) and pregnenediol (5-pregnene-3β,20α-diol) were found to be the most informative discriminators. Although THS was elevated in some adenomas, it was much higher in the carcinoma group. A cut-off of 825 μg/24 h was found to have a sensitivity of 100% and specificity of 99%. In addition, the excretion of unusual metabolites, e.g. 5-pregnene-3α,16α,20α-triol and 5-pregnene-3β,16α,20α-triol, and neonatal metabolites, such as 16α-hydroxypregnenolone (Fig. 15.2), outside the neonatal period were also characteristic of tumours. The retention times of these and other relevant steroids, in terms of their methylene units, is given in Table 15.2.

Ovarian theca lutein cysts may show elevations of the adrenal androgens, DHEA, androsterone and aetiocholanolone as well as the progesterone and 17-hydroxyprogesterone metabolites, pregnanediol and pregnanetriol respectively. There may also be additional 16α-hydroxylated metabolites not usually seen.

Increased androgen excretion was found to be present in 71% cases of carcinoma compared to only 2% of adenoma patients. Excessive excretion of DHEA and metabolites, 16-hydroxyDHEA and androstenetriol, are found in some profiles. Excess DHEA may not necessarily reflect only adrenal steroid production. In one case of isolated DHEA excretion in a female patient initially picked up because of an elevated serum testosterone of 14.3 nmol/L, we found that urine DHEA was approximately three times normal at 3160 μg/24 h (normal <970). No adrenal abnormality was found on imaging and the serum testosterone and urine DHEA suppressed following treatment with the gonadotropin analogue leuprorelin acetate indicating that the androgens were ovarian in origin.

Excessive cortisol production by adenomas has been dealt with in Chap. 16 and will not be further covered here.

Children: Adrenal tumours may present in childhood with the effects of excess androgens, and the urine steroid profile is particularly useful for excluding the

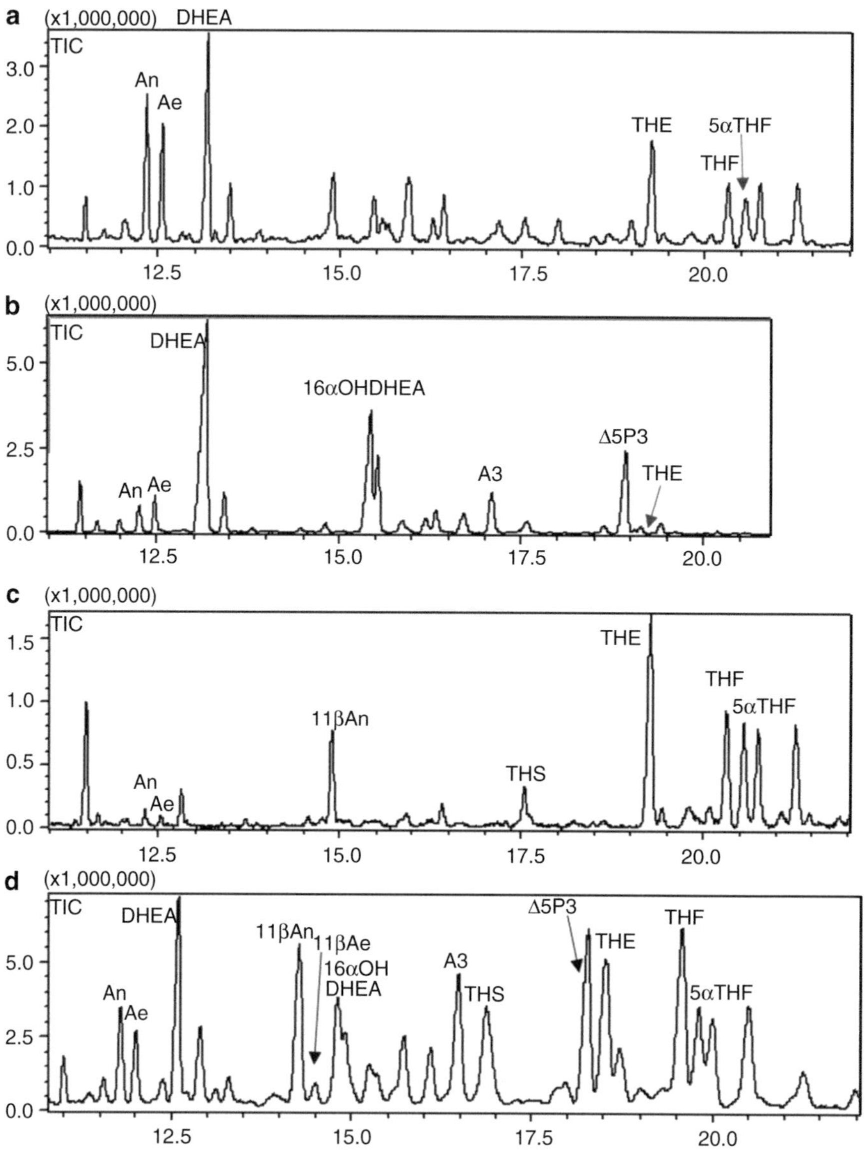

Fig. 15.2 Examples of urine steroid profiles from patients with adrenal adenomas and carcinomas. (**a**) Adrenal androgens predominate; histology consistent with benign adenoma. (**b**) Adrenal tumour expressing increased amounts of Δ5P3, DHEA; cortisol metabolites are suppressed. Histology suggests benign adenoma. (**c**) Sample from a 4-year-old patient subsequently shown to have a benign neoplasm showing increased output of cortisol metabolites (fivefold upper limit of normal). THS is present in this profile, but is not high. (**d**) Profile from patient with an adrenal carcinoma showing excessive output of THS and Δ5P3. Cortisol metabolites are also grossly elevated (tenfold upper limit of normal)

Table 15.2 Steroid metabolites seen in excessive amounts in tumours, retention times (methylene units, MU) of their MO-TMS derivatives and characteristic ions (see appendix for spectra)

Steroid	Trivial name	Retention time (MU)	Relevant ion(s)
5α-Androstan-3α-ol-17-one	Androsterone	25.11	270, 360
5β-Androstan-3α-ol-17-one	Aetiocholanolone	25.28	270, 360
5-Androsten-3β-ol-17-one	Dehydroepiandrosterone (DHEA)	25.75	268, 358
5α-Androstan-3α, 11β-diol-17-one	11β-Androsterone	27.00	448, 358
5-Androsten-3β,16β -diol-17-one	16α-HydroxyDHEA	27.74	266, 446
5-Androsten-3β,16β,17β-triol	Androstenetriol	28.46	432, 329
5β-Pregnane-3α,17α,21-triol-20-one	THS	28.62	564, 474
5-Pregnene-3α,16α,20α-triol		28.62	460, 445
5-Pregnen-3β,16α-diol-20-one	16α-Hydroxypregnenolone	29.38	474
5-Pregnene-3β,17α,20α-triol	Pregnenetriol (Δ5P3)	29.46	433, 253
6β,11β,17,21-Tetrahydroxy-4-pregnene-3,20-dione	6β-Hydroxycortisol	32.73	693, 513

possibility of late-presenting forms of congenital adrenal hyperplasia as a cause of hyperandrogenism. Various patterns of metabolites have been reported including those with excessive DHEA synthesis and those with excessive 11β-hydroxyandrosterone, a metabolite of the adrenal-specific metabolite 11β-hydroxyandrostenedione. In the case of an adrenal tumour, the pattern of abnormal metabolites produced can be used to both monitor the effectiveness of treatment and also recurrence of disease.

15.7 Treatment

Where possible, surgery is the first-line treatment for functional adrenal and gonadal tumours. It is not recommended if asymptomatic, non-functioning and with benign features.

Medical treatments tend to be inhibitors of steroidogenesis or drugs with adrenolytic properties and are primarily used for metastatic disease and as an adjuvant therapy following surgery where there is a high risk of recurrence. The first-line treatment for adrenal carcinoma is mitotane, an adrenolytic drug that is a powerful inducer of CYP3A4 and consequently leads to enhanced cortisol metabolism. As it also causes an increase in cortisol-binding globulin, biochemical evidence of cortisol deficiency may not initially be evident, and concomitant glucocorticoid replacement is essential. Mitotane also causes marked changes to the pattern of metabolites in a urine steroid profile. These changes include a significant increase in the synthesis of 6β-hydroxycortisol (Fig. 15.3) from $<2\%$ of cortisol metabolites in controls to 56% in patients treated with mitotane and hydrocortisone. In addition, the drug inhibits 5α-reductase to a similar degree to that seen following treatment with the

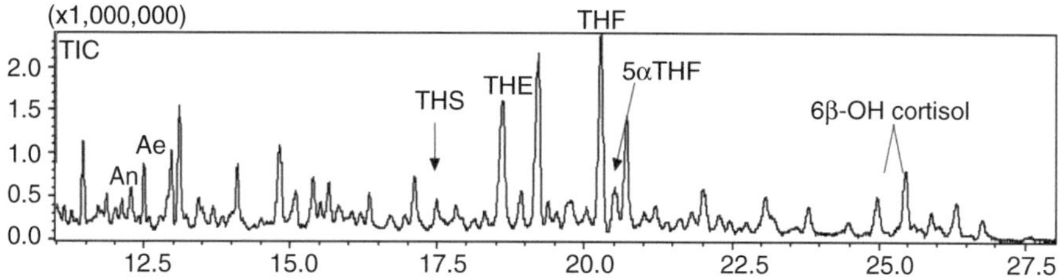

Fig. 15.3 Effect of mitotane on urine steroid profile. Note increased excretion of 6β-hydroxycortisol and reduction of 5αTHF relative to THF. *An* androsterone, *Ae* aetiocholanolone

5α-reductase inhibitor finasteride or in patients with the inherited disorder of steroid 5α-reductase 2 deficiency. The reduction is, however, not as profound for the androsterone/aetiocholanolone pair of 5α/5β metabolites. A reduction in 20β-reduced cortisol metabolites relative to 20α metabolites is also seen, particularly affecting the cortols, cortolones and 6α-hydroxycortolones. Mitotane does not cause inhibition of the steroid 11-hydroxylase enzyme.

Ketoconazole and other antifungal azole drugs are inhibitors of steroidogenesis. This class of drugs typically inhibits several of the steroid biosynthetic steps including 11β- and 17α-hydroxylase enzymes, and the urine steroid profile following such drug treatments may show an increase in, for example, THS and thus may lead to misinterpretation if the analyst is unaware of the treatment regime. As it is markedly hepatotoxic, ketoconazole use is now restricted. Etomidate is another imidazole drug that is an inhibitor of 11β-hydroxylase and the cholesterol side chain cleavage enzyme. It is now mainly used in the critically ill who are unable to take oral treatments. Glucocorticoid excess may also be treated with metyrapone, an inhibitor of 11β-hydroxylase. Its use will lead to an increase in urinary THS, and thus monitoring may be difficult as the 11-deoxycortisol produced may interfere with cortisol measurements if immunoassay is used.

Mifepristone is a glucocorticoid receptor antagonist with a much higher affinity for the receptor than cortisol. As yet there are no adequate parameters to monitor successful treatment with this drug and overtreatment can occur.

Medical treatment for hyperandrogenism includes the anti-androgen drugs cyproterone acetate and spironolactone. The latter is a partial inhibitor of the androgen receptor but is also a competitive inhibitor of the mineralocorticoid receptor and can cause renal dysfunction and hyperkalaemia. Spironolactone can also be used to treat Conn's syndrome prior to surgery. Gonadotrophin analogues can be used to decrease ovarian hyperandrogenism.

Further Reading

Steroid Profiling for Evaluation of Adrenal Neoplasia

Arlt W, Biehl M, Taylor AE, et al. Urine steroid metabolomics as a biomarker tool for detecting malignancy in adrenal tumours. J Clin Endocrinol Metab. 2011;96:3775–84.

Kerkhofs TMA, Kerstens MN, Kema IP, Willems TP, Haak HR. Diagnostic value of urine steroid profiling in the evaluation of adrenal tumours. Horm Canc. 2015;6:168–75.

Tiu SC, Chan AOK, Taylor NF, Lee CY, Loung PY, Choi CH, Shek CC. Use of urinary steroid profiling for diagnosing and monitoring adrenocortical tumours. Hong Kong Med J. 2009;15:463–70.

Management Guidelines

Fassnacht M, Arlt W, Bancos I, et al. Management of adrenal incidentalomas: European Society of Endocrinology Clinical Practice Guideline in collaboration with the European Network for the Study of Adrenal Tumors. Eur J Endocrinol. 2016;175:G1–34.

Cushing's Syndrome 16

Gill Rumsby

16.1 Introduction

Cortisol is required for life. It is a key hormone in the response of the body to hypoglycaemia and other stressors, and its release is regulated by the action of two hormones: the hypothalamic corticotrophin-releasing hormone (CRH) and pituitary adrenocorticotrophic hormone (ACTH) (Fig. 16.1). The negative feedback system that exists in the healthy individual therefore ensures that cortisol is synthesised in response to need and that synthesis is switched off again once the stressful stimulus is over. Cushing's syndrome arises when this regulatory system is overwhelmed either because of an autonomous tumour in the adrenal gland or secondary to excess ACTH either produced by the pituitary (Cushing's disease) or ectopically. The symptoms of Cushing's syndrome include visceral obesity, muscle myopathy, hypertension, insulin resistance, type 2 diabetes mellitus, osteoporosis and hepatic steatosis.

The most common cause of Cushing's syndrome is iatrogenic from the chronic administration of prescription glucocorticoids, in particular topical steroids such as clobetasol and betamethasone for the treatment of psoriasis and eczema or inhaled steroids commonly used for asthma treatment. Some steroid preparations are available over the counter with the potential for excessive usage. It has been estimated that 1% of the population are long-term users of glucocorticoids and of these, approximately two-thirds will suffer some symptoms of glucocorticoid excess.

Endogenous glucocorticoid excess has been estimated to have an incidence in the region of three cases per million inhabitants per year and approximately 0.89 per million per year in children and adolescents. The most common cause of non-iatrogenic Cushing's syndrome is pituitary excess of ACTH (75%), followed by adrenal excess (15%) and ectopic ACTH secretion (less than 1%). Sources of ectopic ACTH include carcinoid tumours in the bronchus, pancreas or thymus,

G. Rumsby
Department of Clinical Biochemistry, University College London Hospitals, London, UK
e-mail: gill.rumsby@nhs.net

G. Rumsby, G. M. Woodward (eds.), *Disorders of Steroidogenesis*,
https://doi.org/10.1007/978-3-319-96364-8_16

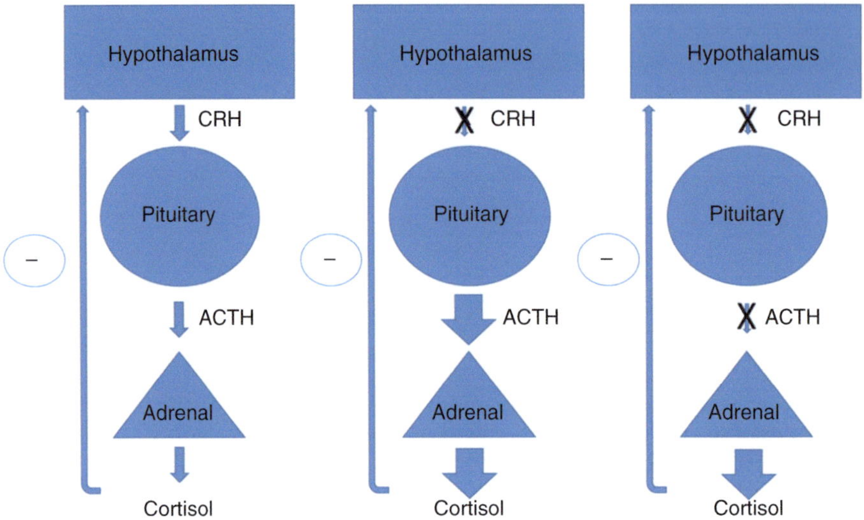

Fig. 16.1 Hypothalamic-pituitary adrenal axis illustrating the negative feedback system controlling cortisol synthesis in a normal subject (left). In pituitary Cushing's syndrome (middle), there is an increase in ACTH (denoted by heavy arrow) leading to increased cortisol production and suppression of CRH. Adrenal Cushing's syndrome will lead to increased cortisol production and suppression of both CRH and ACTH (right)

medullary carcinoma of the thyroid, phaeochromocytoma and small-cell carcinoma of the lungs. Recently it has also been described with a neurofibroma.

The clinical and diagnostic features of Cushing's syndrome are shared by a number of other disorders that can make diagnosis difficult. For example, alcoholism, chronic renal failure and a number of psychiatric disorders including depression may be associated with hypercortisolism – conditions described as pseudo-Cushing's or non-neoplastic (physiologic) Cushing's syndrome. These disorders appear to have effects on the hypothalamus with attenuation of the negative feedback system leading to increased cortisol secretion. It can be difficult to discriminate between these physiologic disorders and Cushing's syndrome itself, with overlap in biochemical testing.

Cushing's syndrome may present progressively, with the patient consulting the GP on a number of occasions with different common conditions, and it may take some time before a unifying diagnosis is made. One study found that the mean time to diagnosis was 6 years. In some cases, the patient may respond poorly to treatment for conditions such as diabetes or hypertension suggesting that there is perhaps a need to investigate more thoroughly. If untreated, Cushing's syndrome has a mortality of 50% at 5 years mainly the result of cardiac failure, myocardial infarction or infection as a result of the immunosuppressive properties of glucocorticoids. The disorder also causes marked morbidity leading to osteoporosis, myopathy, depression and infertility.

The excess cortisol produced in Cushing's syndrome causes profound metabolic changes particularly in adipose tissue. Cortisol is inactivated by the enzyme

11-hydroxysteroid dehydrogenase 2 in the kidney and colon (see Chap. 12) but can be reactivated to cortisol by the enzyme 11β-hydroxysteroid dehydrogenase 1 (11βHSD1) in various tissues, thus enabling interaction with the glucocorticoid receptor. The latter enzyme is widely expressed particularly in the liver, adipose tissue and skeletal muscle and catalyses the conversion of cortisone to cortisol by reduction of the oxo group at carbon 11 to hydroxyl. The reaction is reversible but the reductase reaction is favoured in vivo. Evidence for the role of this enzyme in the Cushing's phenotype comes from patients with hypercortisolism but with no apparent metabolic changes in whom a partial biochemical deficiency of 11βHSD1 could be demonstrated.

16.2 Presentation

The symptoms that are classically associated with Cushing's syndrome and that provide the best discrimination include easy bruising, facial plethora, proximal muscle weakness and purple striae more than 1 cm wide. Other features that may be present include weight gain with central obesity, dorsocervical fat pad (buffalo hump), moon face, menstrual irregularity, diabetes, depression, hypertension and immunosuppression. The disease tends to have an insidious onset in children, obesity occurring in 80% and longitudinal growth retardation in 53%; facial plethora and moon face were found in 83%.

The Endocrine Society guidelines (Nieman et al., 2008) recommend screening for Cushing's syndrome in the following patient groups:

- Patients with unusual features for age, e.g. osteoporosis
- Patients with multiple and progressive features, particularly those associated with Cushing's syndrome (as described above)
- Children with decreasing height centiles and increasing weight
- Patients with adrenal incidentaloma

16.3 Genetics

The exploration of genetic defects arising in tumours is still in its infancy, but a number of genes have been implicated in the pathogenesis of Cushing's syndrome that affect either the functioning of the pituitary corticotrophs or lead to adrenal hyperplasia and carcinoma. In the case of adrenal hyperplasia, these changes mainly affect the cAMP and protein kinase A signalling pathway. One mutation, p.Leu206Arg, in *PRKACA*, the gene encoding the alpha isoform of the catalytic subunit of protein kinase A leads to a gain of function and promotes cell proliferation. This variant was found in the heterozygous state in 37% cases of unilateral adrenocortical adenomas with Cushing's syndrome but not in subclinical Cushing's, the latter defined as at least one abnormal biochemical test but with no catabolic features of the disease. Germ line mutations were associated with bilateral hyperplasia, whereas somatic mutations, i.e. found only in the tumour, were associated with unilateral disease. The majority of tumours are sporadic, but 5–10% of cases will have an inherited predisposition, e.g. Li-Fraumeni syndrome, multiple endocrine neoplasia type 1, Lynch syndrome, Beckwith-Wiedemann syndrome and familial adenomatous polyposis.

Mutations in *USP8*, the gene encoding ubiquitin-specific protease 8 protein, have been found in 40% of pituitary corticotroph adenomas. This protein inhibits lysosomal degradation of epidermal growth factor receptor (EGFR), and the gain of function mutations lead to increased deubiquitination of EGFR, and consequently it is rescued from degradation. The process leads to induction of proopiomelanocortin transcription and ACTH secretion. Approximately 5–10% of cases of multiple endocrine neoplasia type 1 with mutations in *MENIN* have pituitary tumours producing excess ACTH.

The majority of paediatric adrenocortical carcinomas have mutations in *TP53*, a tumour suppressor gene. The findings in tumours are further covered in Chap. 15.

16.4 Diagnosis

The recommended approach for the biochemical diagnosis of Cushing's syndrome is provided in the Endocrine Society guidelines (Nieman et al., 2008), although this strategy is still not fully adopted.

Initial investigation should use one of the following initial tests:

- 1 mg overnight dexamethasone suppression test (DST)
- Longer low-dose DST (2 mg/day for 48 h)
- Urine free cortisol (UFC; at least two measurements)
- Late-night salivary cortisol (two measurements)

These tests assess three different aspects of cortisol physiology: firstly, reduced sensitivity to glucocorticoid negative feedback assessed by low-dose dexamethasone suppression testing; secondly, increased production of cortisol as assessed by 24-h UFC measurement; and, thirdly, failure of the normal diurnal rhythm of cortisol tested by measurement of late-night salivary cortisol.

The overnight dexamethasone suppression test with measurement of serum cortisol the following morning is by far the easiest to carry out in a GP setting requiring no specialist methodology. In the case of Cushing's syndrome and also pseudo-Cushing's syndrome, there will be no suppression of cortisol. There is, however, some difficulty in deciding an appropriate cut-off, and this will also depend on the assay although in most cases a normal response would usually involve suppression of serum cortisol to less than 50 nmol/L. Care also needs to be taken to ensure that the patient is not taking any drugs that induce the CYP3A4 enzyme, e.g. any common anticonvulsants including phenobarbitone and carbamazepine, as this may lead to increased metabolism of dexamethasone and thus inadequate suppression giving a false result.

Measurement of UFC requires a 24-h urine collection, and instructions need to be given to the patient on exactly how to do this to avoid under- and over-collection that will impact on interpretation of results. The test measures cortisol that has not been metabolised in the body. This fraction normally constitutes only a small percentage (2–3%) of the total cortisol metabolites but can be much higher in Cushing's syndrome provided there is no renal impairment – UFC decreases when creatinine clearance is less than 60 mL/min. Again, there are problems with measurement. Immunoassay is prone to interference from other steroids although ironically this may actually make the test more useful than the more specific LC-MS methods, particularly in the case of adrenal tumours. The recommended cut-off for a positive test is above the upper limit of normal for the laboratory, assuming that a complete collection has been received. The high biological variability (intrapatient coefficient of variation of 50%), and problems with collection, means that it is recommended to repeat on more than one occasion. False negatives can also occur particularly in cyclical Cushing's syndrome, and in such cases the patient should be instructed to collect samples following a symptomatic episode.

Salivary cortisol provides another means of measuring free, unmetabolised, cortisol. As concentrations of cortisol in this medium are low (<10 nmol/L), the accuracy and imprecision of the methodology are important. There is lack of standardisation of methods and therefore considerable variation in reference ranges that makes the assignment of a common cut-off impossible at the moment.

For a negative test in a patient with a low index of suspicion for Cushing's syndrome, the recommendation is to review in 6 months if symptoms progress. A negative test result in a patient with high index of suspicion and those cases with positive test results should be followed up with one of the other tests and then referred to an endocrinologist for further assessment.

Pseudo-Cushing's syndrome may give positive results in screening tests. It is recommended that this is excluded by the performance of a dexamethasone suppression test combined with CRH stimulation (DST-CRH). The rationale for this test is that those patients with a physiological cause of hypercortisolism retain sensitivity to glucocorticoid suppression and there will be no effect of CRH on stimulation of ACTH and cortisol. By contrast, those with Cushing's show an increase in ACTH and cortisol.

Subclinical Cushing's syndrome is the term given to those patients who exhibit autonomous cortisol secretion without the obvious stigmata of Cushing's syndrome. They may, however, exhibit some of the adverse effects of chronic glucocorticoid excess including diabetes, hypertension and osteoporosis. The presence of autonomous secretion in these cases appears to be best demonstrated by failure to suppress serum cortisol with 1 mg dexamethasone followed by one or more of the tests listed above.

16.5 Case Study

A 26-year-old female presented to the GP with a history of extensive and painful genital warts. On examination, she was found to have purple tinged skin on her legs, stretch marks around the thighs and hips, hair loss and low mood.

Serum cortisol failed to suppress after dexamethasone (cortisol 650 nmol/L). Following referral to an endocrinologist, further tests, including UFC, salivary cortisol and imaging, were performed.

UFC was >800 nmol/L (normal <248), and late-night salivary cortisol on two consecutive nights was 44.7 and 51.8 nmol/L (>8.6 suggests Cushing's syndrome), all results consistent with Cushing's syndrome. A urine steroid profile showed the characteristic profile of excess cortisol metabolites suggestive of a cortisol-producing adenoma. There was no excess of intermediates to indicate carcinoma. A mass on the left adrenal was visible on MRI. Following unilateral adrenalectomy, the patient showed rapid symptom improvement.

16.6 Steroid Profile

A urine steroid profile is not usually one of the tests used for the investigation of pituitary hypercortisolism but can be particularly helpful if the cause is suspected to be an adrenal source – the pattern of metabolites providing some discrimination between adenoma and carcinoma (see Chap. 15). A 24-h urine sample is preferable for this analysis as misleading results can otherwise occur in, e.g. a particularly concentrated random sample taken in the middle of the day when cortisol metabolite excretion is maximal.

Total cortisol metabolites are typically increased (median 34.0 mg/day, range 13.3–327) in Cushing's syndrome compared with 6.1 (range 2.5–10.3 mg/day) in controls, secondary to an increase in the cortisol secretion rate. In the case of an adrenal cortisol-producing tumour, adrenal androgen metabolites, androsterone and aetiocholanolone, may be lower than expected because the cortisol produced by the hyperplastic adrenal leads to suppression of pituitary ACTH. The profile will also typically show an excess of cortisol relative to cortisone metabolites, reflecting the inability of 11HSD2 enzyme to metabolise the excess cortisol to cortisone (Fig. 16.2), possibly reflecting substrate excess or product inhibition of the enzyme. This situation leads to an increased (THF + 5αTHF)/THE ratio with values of 1.81 (mean, range 1.09–9.99) reported in Cushing's syndrome versus 0.81 (range 0.51–1.47) in controls. In the case of Cushing's syndrome arising from ectopic ACTH

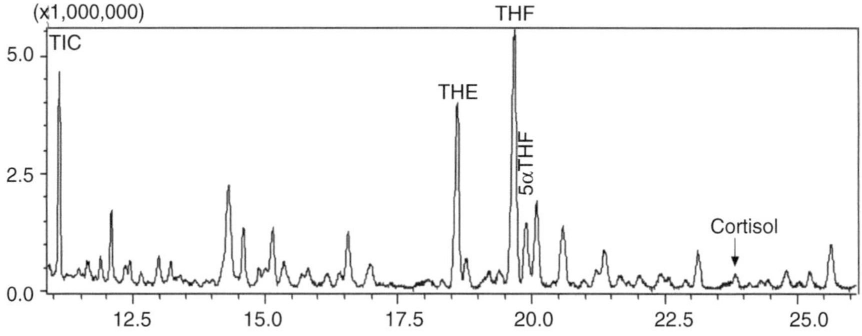

Fig. 16.2 Typical profile from patient with Cushing's syndrome arising from an adrenal adenoma. Note the overall increase in cortisol output with an excess of cortisol to cortisone metabolites, decreased 5αTHF and the presence of free cortisol

Table 16.1 Steroid metabolites used for assessment of Cushing's syndrome, retention times (methylene units, MU) of their MO-TMS derivatives and characteristic ions (see appendix for spectra)

Systematic name	Steroid	MU	Relevant ions
3α-Hydroxy-5α-androstan-17-one	Androsterone (An)	25.11	270, 360
3α-Hydroxy-5β-androstan-17-one	Aetiocholanolone (Ae)	25.28	270, 360
3α,17α,21-Trihydroxy-5β-pregnan-11,20-one	Tetrahydrocortisone (THE)	29.65	578, 488
3α,11β,21-Trihydroxy-5β-pregnan-20-one	Tetrahydrocorticosterone (THB)	30.00	188, 564
3α,11β,17α,21-Trihydroxy-5β-pregnan-20-one	Tetrahydrocortisol (THF)	30.24	652, 472
3α,11β,17α,21-Trihydroxy-5α-pregnan-20-one	α-Tetrahydrocortisol (αTHF)	30.39	652, 472
5β-Pregnane-3α,11β,17α,20α,21-pentol	α-Cortol	31.20	523, 343
11β,17α,21-Trihydroxy-4-pregnene-3,20-dione	Cortisol	32.54/32.83	605, 515

secretion, these values can be even higher. There is also suppression of 5α-reductase activity leading to a characteristic decrease in the 5αTHF/THF ratio. Free cortisol may also be clearly visible in the profile.

Linear discriminant analysis has shown that the following steroids act as useful biomarkers for Cushing's syndrome: higher concentrations of tetrahydrocorticosterone, THF, 5αTHF and α-cortol as well as lower tetrahydrocortisone when compared to controls and patients with non-functioning adrenal incidentalomas. The retention times of these and other relevant components are given in Table 16.1.

16.7 Treatment

Treatment depends on the underlying cause of Cushing's syndrome, but for all non-iatrogenic causes, surgery is the primary approach. For iatrogenic disease, the drug treatment must be tapered off; sudden cessation is not recommended because adrenal suppression may have occurred and thus an adrenal crisis may be precipitated.

Transsphenoidal surgery can provide a cure in approximately 80% of patients with a pituitary tumour, while either unilateral or bilateral adrenalectomy is the preferred approach for an adrenal cause of Cushing's syndrome.

Dopamine and somatostatin receptors have been identified as targets for medical treatment of pituitary adenomas. Some 80% of pituitary adenomas express dopamine receptors subtype 2 and may therefore be responsive to cabergoline, a dopamine agonist. Pasireotide binds to somatostatin receptors, particularly to the sst5 receptor subtype expressed in pituitary adenomas and has been shown to suppress cortisol in about one-fifth of patients but at the expense of worsening glucose tolerance.

Medical treatments directed at cortisol synthesis include adrenolytic agents, e.g. mitotane; steroid synthesis blockers including ketoconazole, metyrapone and etomidate; and the glucocorticoid receptor blocker, mifepristone. Mitotane, metyrapone and ketoconazole can all alter steroid metabolism and lead to abnormal-looking urine steroid profiles. Mitotane increases cortisol metabolism and also causes an abnormal 5αTHF/THF ratio similar to that seen with finasteride treatment. Metyrapone inhibits 11β-hydroxylase and therefore there is an increase in THS excretion. Ketoconazole and etomidate both inhibit 11β-hydroxylase and some of the other enzymes in the pathway. As the treatment regime is often not documented on requests for urine steroid profile, it is important that one keeps in mind these effects to avoid errors in interpretation of an apparently abnormal profile. Additional detail on this aspect is given in Chap. 15.

Further Reading

Genetics

Albani A, Theodoropoulou M, Reincke M. Genetics of Cushing's disease. Clin Endocrinol. 2018;88:3–12.

Biochemical Diagnosis

El Farhan N, Rees DA, Evans C. Measuring cortisol in serum, urine and saliva—are our assays good enough? Ann Clin Biochem. 2016;54:308–22.

Kotłowska A, Puzyn T, Sworczak K, Stepnowski P, Szefer P. Metabolomic biomarkers in urine of Cushing's syndrome patients. Int J Mol Sci. 2017;18:294.

Endocrinology

Nieman LK, Biller BMK, Findling JW, Newell-Price J, Savage MO, Stewart PM, Montori VM. The diagnosis of Cushing's syndrome: an endocrine society clinical practice guideline. J Clin Endocrinol Metab. 2008;93:1526–40.

Tomlinson JW, Draper N, Mackie J, Johnson AP, Holder G, Wood P, Stewart PM. Absence of Cushingoid phenotype in a patient with Cushing's disease due to defective cortisone to cortisol conversion. J Clin Endocrinol Metab. 2002;87:57–62.

Effect of Mitotane on Steroid Profile

Ghataore L, Chakraborti I, Aylwin SJ, Schulte KM, Dworakowska D, Coskeran P, Taylor NF. Effects of mitotane treatment on human steroid metabolism: implications for patient management. Endocr Connect. 2012;1:37–47.

17 Adrenal Insufficiency

Gill Rumsby

17.1 Introduction

Adrenal insufficiency is the name given to a failure of cortisol synthesis from whatever cause. The symptoms of insufficiency can include chronic fatigue, muscle weakness, vomiting, low blood pressure precipitating dizziness or fainting and weight loss. In addition, when the cause is adrenal failure itself, i.e. primary disease, the normal negative feedback from the adrenal gland is lifted, and adrenocorticotrophic hormone (ACTH) secretion is stimulated. This hormone is produced by cleavage of the pro-opiomelanocortin (POMC) peptide, and there is an associated increase in production of the melanocyte-stimulating hormone (αMSH) cleaved from the same POMC precursor. Thus, there is a tendency to get darkening of the skin as a result of excessive secretion of αMSH.

Secondary adrenal failure is the result of ACTH deficiency either because of disease, e.g. a tumour, or from failure of ACTH synthesis or action. Tertiary adrenal insufficiency arises from deficiency of the hypothalamic corticotrophin-releasing hormone (CRH). The causes of these disorders will be dealt with separately.

In general, genetic disorders more commonly present in childhood, while acquired forms are more prevalent in adults.

17.1.1 Primary Adrenal Insufficiency

Primary adrenal insufficiency (PAI) can occur as a result of developmental failure, drug treatment, infection, autoimmunity and the inheritance of disorders affecting adrenal steroid biosynthesis. It is rare with a prevalence of 93–100 per million.

G. Rumsby
Department of Clinical Biochemistry, University College London Hospitals, London, UK
e-mail: gill.rumsby@nhs.net

G. Rumsby, G. M. Woodward (eds.), *Disorders of Steroidogenesis*,
https://doi.org/10.1007/978-3-319-96364-8_17

The most common cause of adrenal insufficiency, accounting for 68–94% cases, is autoimmune adrenalitis, first described by Thomas Addison in the late nineteenth century. This disorder leads to destruction of adrenal tissue. Isolated adrenal insufficiency accounts for 30–40% cases of adrenalitis, while the remainder may be part of the autoimmune polyglandular syndromes (APS) of which the most common is APS type 2. APS type 1, accounting for 30–40% of cases, is found in association with hypoparathyroidism and chronic mucocutaneous candidiasis and arises as a result of mutations in the autoimmune regulator protein (AIRE). This protein plays a key role in presenting tissue-specific self-antigens to naïve T cells in the thymus leading to the negative selection of self-reacting T-cells. The disorder is also characterised by antibodies to interferon (INF)-ω (sensitivity 99%) and INF-α 2 (sensitivity 91%).

APS type 2 (50–60% of APS cases) has adrenal insufficiency and either autoimmune thyroid disease (69% of APS2 cases), type 1 diabetes (52%) or both (12%) and has been associated with mutations in cytotoxic T-lymphocyte-associated protein 4 (CTLA-4) and with particular HLA-DR3 and HLA-DR4 haplotypes. APS type 3 has autoimmune thyroid disease but normal adrenal function, while type 4 has adrenal insufficiency and other autoimmune disorders but normal thyroid function.

The adrenal glands tend to be small in adrenalitis and in active disease contain mononuclear cell infiltrate. Autoimmune adrenal disease is characterised by the presence of adrenal antibodies in the serum of patients, primarily directed at the 21-hydroxylase enzyme, but other enzymes of the steroid pathway may also be targets.

In the absence of adrenal autoantibodies, one must consider alternative causes of PAI (Fig. 17.1). Infection, including tuberculosis and HIV, is the next most common underlying pathology. Hypoadrenalism as a result of surgery or medication (ketoconazole, mitotane, metyrapone, etidomate) should be obvious from the patient

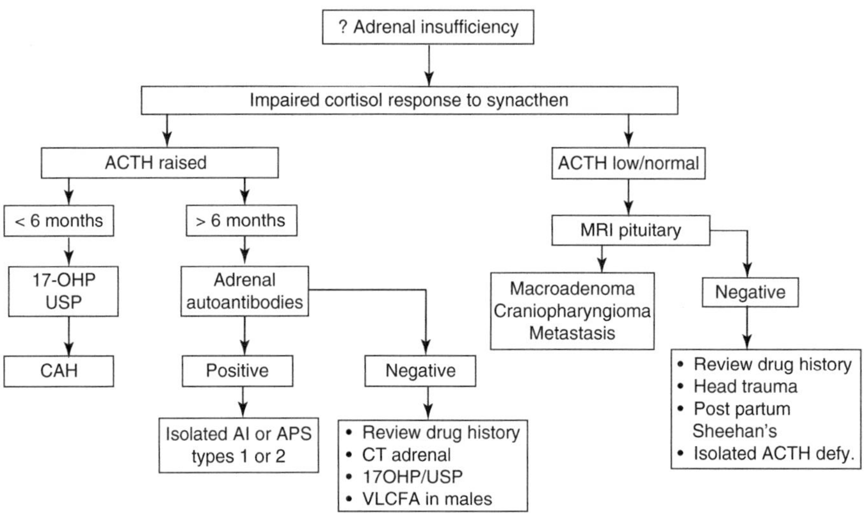

Fig. 17.1 Investigation of adrenal insufficiency. *17OHP* 17-hydroxyprogesterone, *USP* urine steroid profile, *VLCFA* very long chain fatty acids

history. The recent adoption of abiraterone, an inhibitor of the 17α-hydroxylase enzyme (see Chap. 7), for the treatment of prostate cancer requires concomitant hydrocortisone replacement; otherwise adrenal failure ensues. Prednisolone can also induce adrenal failure, and should be tapered off or consideration given to hydrocortisone cover on cessation of treatment. It should also be remembered that the use of drugs that induce CYP3A4, e.g. phenytoin, can increase metabolism of cortisol leading to insufficiency. Adrenal haemorrhage as a cause of adrenal insufficiency can be investigated by CT scan.

Genetic causes of PAI include congenital adrenal hyperplasia; early disorders of steroid biosynthesis, e.g. Smith-Lemli-Opitz syndrome; adrenoleukodystrophy; developmental defects resulting from mutations in transcription factors, e.g. steroidogenic factor 1 (SF-1); and familial glucocorticoid deficiency. These conditions will need to be investigated using a variety of biochemical tests including urine steroid profiles and in some cases will require confirmation by molecular genetics. The most common genetic cause is congenital adrenal hyperplasia arising from steroid 21-hydroxylase deficiency. This disorder and the other forms of CAH are dealt with in their relevant chapters in this book. Primary adrenal insufficiency also affects aldosterone synthesis and is therefore accompanied by renal salt losing and an elevated renin. Exceptions to this are the rare non-salt losing forms of congenital adrenal hyperplasia, e.g. 11- and 17α-hydroxylase deficiencies, that leave the aldosterone pathway unimpaired.

Adrenoleukodystrophy is an X-linked disorder with variable phenotype. It is caused by mutations in the ATP-binding cassette subfamily D member 1 (*ABCD1*) gene that encodes the adrenoleukodystrophy protein (ALDP) needed to transfer fatty acids into the peroxisomes. Adrenal insufficiency may be accompanied by delayed development, progressive stiffness and weakness as a result of adrenomyeloneuropathy. Females may occasionally be affected reflecting inactivation of the X-chromosome.

The orphan nuclear receptor 0B1 (*NR0B1*, formerly known as DAX1) is a dominant negative regulator of transcription. Its exact role in development is unclear, but it is essential for the development of the adrenal, hypothalamus, pituitary, ovary and testis. Mutations in the *NR0B1* gene can cause X-linked congenital adrenal hypoplasia and hypogonadotropic hypogonadism. More than 60% present in the first weeks of life with PAI, either with hypoglycaemia or renal salt loss. Some may present later with delayed or arrested puberty.

Familial glucocorticoid deficiency is an autosomal recessive group of disorders. There are at least three genes involved, two of which affect the ACTH receptor. The first of these, *MRC2*, encodes the ACTH receptor, and mutations either prevent movement of the receptor to the cell membrane or its interaction with ACTH in the membrane. The ACTH receptor is activated by the melanocortin 2 receptor accessory protein (MRAP), and mutations in this protein impair transport of the receptor to the cell membrane. The third gene product is the mitochondrial enzyme nicotinamide nucleotide transhydrogenase (NNT). Mutations in NNT lead to impaired NADPH production, an increase in reactive oxygen species and cell death ultimately leading to impaired glucocorticoid production.

17.1.2 Secondary Adrenal Insufficiency

Secondary adrenal insufficiency is more common than primary with a prevalence of 150–280 per million and includes any factor affecting the production of ACTH. In contrast to PAI, renal salt losing is not a feature of secondary disease as the synthesis of aldosterone, regulated by the renin-angiotensin-aldosterone axis, is unimpaired. The most common causes do not usually lead to ACTH loss in isolation but as part of a generalised loss of pituitary function in which ACTH is often the last hormone to go. Pituitary macroadenoma, defined as a benign growth >1 cm in size, is the most frequent cause of secondary PAI. These growths possibly exert their affect by compression of the portal vessels of the pituitary stalk. Craniopharyngiomas are the third most common intracranial tumour, and these and meningiomas can also cause pituitary insufficiency. Infection, e.g. tuberculosis and infiltration by granulomatous disease, e.g. sarcoidosis or histiocytosis, and pituitary apoplexy can all lead to pan-hypopituitarism. Brain damage following surgery or radiation can cause pituitary failure particularly affecting growth hormone secretion. ACTH, unlike growth hormone, is not particularly sensitive to radiation damage requiring radiation dosage in excess of 30 Gy before loss of anterior pituitary function is seen. Finally, exogenous glucocorticoid use causes atrophy of the pituitary corticotrophs; thus cessation of treatment should be done with care to avoid precipitating an adrenal crisis.

There are some rare, monogenic causes of ACTH deficiency. Combined pituitary hormone deficiencies (CPHD) particularly CPHD 2, 4, 5 and 6 are disorders caused by mutations in the genes *PROP1*, *LHX4*, *HESX1* and *OTX2*, respectively, encoding transcription factors affecting pituitary development. In some cases pituitary function may be initially normal and declines with age. The clinical phenotypes are very variable ranging from normal height to severe growth retardation and a range of craniofacial and midline defects of development. Isolated ACTH deficiency can be caused as the result of mutations in T box 19 transcription factor (TBX19) required for the initiation of transcription of the POMC gene. Some mutations have also been shown in the POMC gene that lead to secondary adrenal insufficiency. The phenotype of patients with defects in POMC and TBX19 is similar having features of adrenal insufficiency, obesity and red hair, although as more patients are described red hair does not appear to be an invariant finding.

Triple A deficiency (Allgrove syndrome) is a disorder affecting the autonomic nervous system characterised by achalasia, Addison's disease and alacrima (lack of tears), the latter often being the first sign of the disease. It is caused by mutations in ALADIN, a nuclear pore protein that plays a role in the movement of molecules into and out of the nucleus. It is not yet clear how lack of this protein causes triple A syndrome.

17.1.3 Tertiary Adrenal Insufficiency

The most common cause of tertiary adrenal insufficiency is exogenous steroid use suppressing the release of CRH.

17.2 Presentation

Adrenal insufficiency can present in a variety of ways depending on the severity and underlying cause. Symptoms of primary adrenal failure include abdominal pain, nausea and vomiting, postural hypotension and, in cases of acute electrolyte abnormalities, fitting.

Acute secondary adrenal insufficiency may present with a sudden onset headache. Chronic disease will often have rather non-specific symptoms and reflect the particular pituitary hormones affected but may include hypogonadism or hypothyroidism.

17.3 Genetics

The vast majority of cases of adrenal insufficiency are acquired disorders, but mutations in a surprisingly large number of genes can also give rise to PAI. These are too numerous to detail in this chapter, and the more common disorders only will be mentioned but others are described in a recent review (Flück, 2017), and the genetics of the steroid biosynthetic disorders are covered in their individual chapters.

A number of mutations in *AIRE* have been described in patients with APS1 of which there are two relatively common changes described in North America and Europe: c.769C>T change in exon 6 causing a nonsense change, p.Arg257*, and a 13 base pair deletion in exon 8, c.967_979delCTGTCCCCTCCGC leading to a frame shift mutation, p.Leu323SerfsX51. This disorder has autosomal recessive inheritance.

In some cases PAI can be the result of syndromic disorders. One particular disorder, X-linked adrenal hypoplasia congenita, can arise from isolated mutations in *NR0B1*, a coregulator of transcription for SF1, but it can also arise from a contiguous gene deletion of *NR0B1* with the genes for Duchenne muscular dystrophy and glycerol kinase deficiency. Thus the phenotype can be quite variable depending on the size of the deletion. Duplication of *NR0B1* can give rise to 46XY sex reversal.

Genetic causes of secondary adrenal insufficiency include mutations in *POMC*, and a number of these have been described. One mutation of particular interest is a missense change p.Arg8Cys that is part of both ACTH and α-MSH peptides. The mutation does not affect the immunoreactivity of the peptides and thus the hormone appears elevated in biochemical assays, but it is biologically inactive. Mutations in *POMC* are inherited as autosomal recessive disorders although there is some suggestion that heterozygosity for *POMC* variants may have an influence on body size.

17.4 Diagnosis

Any patient presenting with otherwise unexplained potential symptoms of Addison's disease should be assessed for adrenal failure. Routine electrolytes may show the characteristic hyperkalaemia and hyponatraemia picture along with disproportionally raised urea if the patient is dehydrated.

The essential test for assessment of adrenal function is measurement of cortisol and ACTH in a blood sample. Cortisol and ACTH both have a significant diurnal variation with the peak in the morning around 08.30 and nadir between 24.00 and 01.00. As total cortisol is routinely measured, the interpretation of results can be affected by any factors affecting cortisol-binding globulin (CBG). This protein binds approximately 80–90% of cortisol, and consequently any increase or decrease of CBG will have an effect on the total cortisol measured. Oral oestrogens and pregnancy are the main factors to be considered here, both leading to increased CBG. In addition, there is considerable variation in cortisol assays, and historical cut-offs indicating adrenal sufficiency may no longer apply. Instead, the onus is on each laboratory to develop their own cut-offs to exclude adrenal insufficiency.

The initial assessment for Addison's disease should ideally be done by measuring serum cortisol at 08.00–09.00, random results being of limited use. In general a value of cortisol greater than 600 nmol/L at any time excludes Addison's disease, while a value less than 100 nmol/L at 08.00–09.00 might be considered deficient and require further investigation.

Stimulation of the adrenal glands with either high-dose (250 μg) or low-dose (1 μg) corticotrophin (also known as a Synacthen test) given either intravenously or intramuscularly is used to assess adrenal insufficiency. There does not appear to be any difference in the two regimes in terms of diagnostic accuracy, but there is considerable variation between laboratories in terms of time of testing post dose (30 or 60 min) and the cut-off used, the latter of course affected by the local cortisol assay.

A plasma ACTH measurement taken around 08.00–09.00 of more than twofold the upper limit for the assay in the presence of an inappropriately low cortisol is also supportive of primary adrenal failure. Renin is also elevated in PAI in the presence of a low aldosterone. More specific tests would then be required to define the cause of PAI and may include a urine steroid profile and 17-hydroxyprogesterone if congenital adrenal hyperplasia is suspected from the age of the patient and/or additional symptoms, e.g. hyperandrogenism. Alternatively adrenal antibodies may be the next step (Fig. 17.1).

If secondary adrenal insufficiency, one would expect both ACTH and cortisol to be reduced. Adrenal reserve can still be assessed by Synacthen stimulation as the acute response to Synacthen in those with chronic ACTH deficiency is impaired, but this response does take time to develop so may not be helpful, for example, immediately after surgery in someone suspected of pituitary failure. The high-dose Synacthen test has a poorer sensitivity for secondary disease (64% versus 92% for PAI) and is therefore useful to rule in adrenal insufficiency but if negative does not rule it out. Further investigation of the hypothalamic-pituitary axis can take the form of an insulin tolerance test that also assesses growth hormone reserve. This dynamic function test is regarded as the gold standard, but it can be dangerous requiring close medical supervision and cannot be used on patients with a history of seizures or cardiac disease or the elderly. The glucagon stimulation test may be used instead which measures the response of cortisol and GH although it is not clear if the response is to the nausea induced by the glucagon or to the rise and fall of glucose.

CRH stimulation (100 μg synthetic CRH i.v.) is possible with subsequent measurement of ACTH and can be used to investigate suspected isolated ACTH deficiency but is rarely used.

17.5 Case Study

A 45-year-old man presented to the emergency department with a history of vomiting and lethargy. He was a known type 1 diabetic. Routine serum electrolytes on admission showed the following:

Sodium	123 mmol/L	(135–145)
Potassium	6.8 mmol/L	(3.5–4.5)
Urea	18.0 mmol/L	(2.5–7.8)
Creatinine	246 μmol/L	(80–115)

Serum cortisol was added to the original request and was low at 26 nmol/L (>415 nmol/L at 09.00). The sample had been taken late in the afternoon so a Synacthen test was carried out prior to initiation of glucocorticoid. There was essentially no rise in serum cortisol after 30 min (250–300 nmol/L) confirming a diagnosis of adrenal insufficiency. The patient was also found to be hypothyroid (TSH 26 IU/L, ref. range <5) and a diagnosis of APS type 2 made.

17.6 Steroid Profile

The most common cause of adrenal insufficiency in the neonate is congenital adrenal hyperplasia of which 21-hydroxylase deficiency is the most common. Thus measurement of serum 17-hydroxyprogesterone is a useful preliminary test in conjunction with a urine steroid profile to look for this and other forms of CAH in a single urine sample taken prior to commencement of treatment. Typical neonatal profiles for the different disorders of CAH are described in the individual chapters in this book.

These disorders can also present in later life although usually with symptoms of hyperandrogenism developing in response to the high ACTH drive needed to maintain normal glucocorticoid output. Serum cortisol response to Synacthen stimulation is typically impaired but may equivocal with values at the lower end of normal. It is therefore essential to also measure the response of 17-hydroxyprogesterone to Synacthen along with a urine steroid profile (off treatment) to pick up abnormal metabolites.

Adrenal hypoplasia in the first few days of life demonstrates a profile with almost complete absence of the 3β-hydroxy-5-ene steroids consistent with hypoplasia of the fetal zone of the adrenal gland. The main steroids produced are identical to the glucuronide fraction of the normal neonate, i.e. with tetrahydrocortisone and 6α-hydroxytetrahydrocortisone as the dominant cortisol metabolites. This pattern is also seen in the anencephalic newborn, one of the causes of low maternal oestriol excretion in the third trimester. Progesterone metabolites, e.g. 6α-hydroxypregnanolone, 16α-hydroxypregnanolone and 5β-pregnane-3α,16α,20α-triol, are also present. These are largely placental in origin (Table 17.1).

In the case of complete failure of the adrenal glands, the pattern of steroids would be normal, but the output would be much reduced. This situation is more difficult to interpret in the case of a random sample without some measure of urine concentration, e.g. creatinine.

Adrenal suppression as a result of prednisolone treatment is illustrated in Fig. 17.2. In this profile almost all endogenous steroids are significantly reduced, but prednisolone metabolites are evident.

Table 17.1 Metabolites of relevant steroids, retention times (methylene units, MU) of their MO-TMS derivatives and characteristic ions (see appendix for spectra)

Systematic name	Trivial name	MU	Relevant ions
5β-Pregnan-3α,6α-diol-20-one	6α-Hydroxypregnanolone	28.52	388, 298
5β-Pregnan-3α,16α-diol-20-one	16α-Hydroxypregnanolone	28.52	386, 188
5β-Pregnan-3α,16α,20α-triol		29.38	462, 117
5β-Pregnan-3α,17α,21-triol-11,20-dione	THE	29.65	578, 488
5β-Pregnan-3α,6α,17α,21-tetrol-11,20-dione	6α OH THE	30.80	666, 576
Drug metabolites			
3α,11β,17,21-Tetrahydroxy-5β-pregnane-1,20-dione	Tetrahydroprednisolone	30.37	650, 560
	6β-Hydroxyprednisolone peak 1	33.00	632, 219
	20-Hydroxyprednisolone peak 1	33.25	677, 335
	6β-Hydroxyprednisolone peak 2	33.27	632, 219
	20-Hydroxyprednisolone peak 2	33.40	677, 335

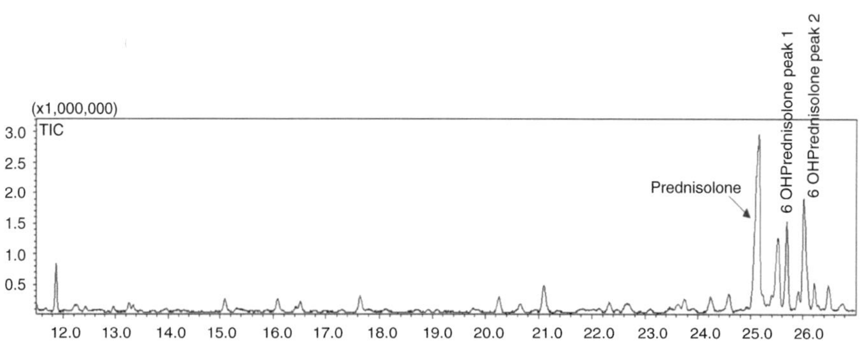

Fig. 17.2 Urine steroid profile from patient on prednisolone showing the characteristic urinary metabolites of this drug and the complete suppression of all normal adrenal steroids

17.7 Treatment

Adrenal insufficiency regardless of cause is treated by glucocorticoid replacement with additional mineralocorticoids if aldosterone synthesis is also impaired. The Endocrine Society guidelines recommend hydrocortisone or cortisone acetate in three divided doses per day. Prednisolone, administered once or twice a day, can be used as an alternative, but dexamethasone is not recommended because of difficulties titrating the dose and the risk of Cushing's side effects. Treatment should be monitored clinically by assessing, e.g. weight and blood pressure. Secondary adrenal insufficiency may require additional hormone replacement including thyroxine, growth hormone and gonadal steroids.

Further Reading

Diagnosis

Bornstein SR, Allolio B, Arlt W, Barthel A, Don-Wauchope A, et al. Diagnosis and treatment of primary adrenal insufficiency: an Endocrine Society clinical practice guideline. J Clin Endocrinol Metab. 2016;101:364–89.

El-Farhan N, Rees DA, Evans C. Measuring cortisol in serum, urine and saliva—are our assays good enough? Ann Clin Biochem. 2017;54:308–22.

Grossman AB. The diagnosis and management of central hypoadrenalism. J Clin Endocrinol Metab. 2010;95:4855–63.

Pathophysiology and Genetics

Flück CE. Update on pathogenesis of primary adrenal insufficiency: beyond steroid enzyme deficiency and autoimmune adrenal destruction. Eur J Endocrinol. 2017;177:R99–111.

Johnson MB, Hattersley AT, Flanagan SE. Monogenic autoimmune diseases of the endocrine system. Lancet Diabetes Endocrinol. 2016;4:862–72.

Appendix: Common Steroid Identification—GC-MS Mass Spectra

Gary Woodward, Francis Lam, and Gill Rumsby

As described in Chap. 3, steroid profiling in the context of steroidogenic conditions is performed by GC-MS analysis following conjugate hydrolysis and derivatisation. Below are the mass spectra used for identification of urine steroids described throughout this book, and compiled during routine practice within our laboratory. Steroids are given in approximate order of their retention times.

Androstanediol (internal standard)

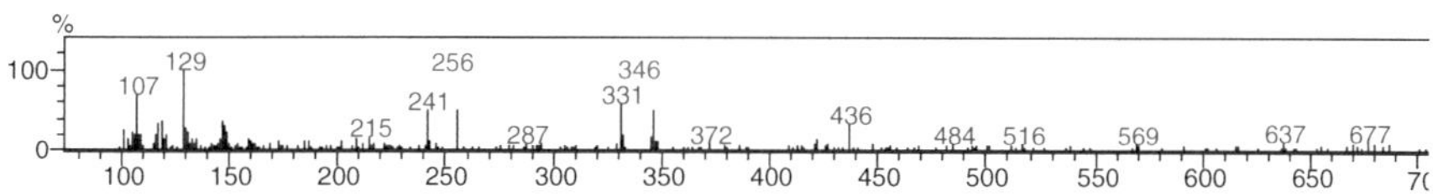

Pregnadienol

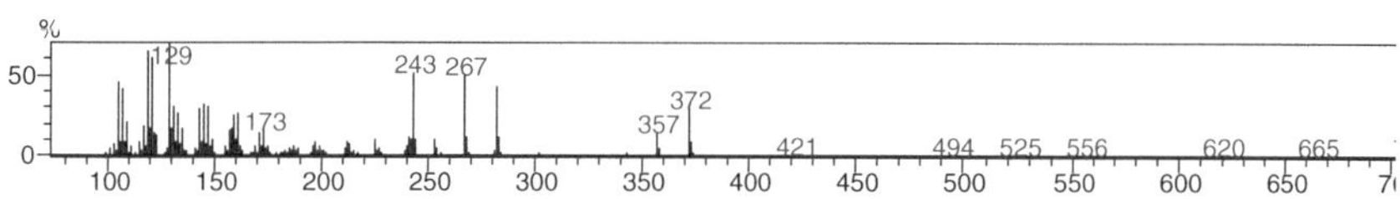

G. Woodward · G. Rumsby
Department of Clinical Biochemistry, University College London Hospitals, London, UK

F. Lam
Level 2-Chemistry, Health Services Laboratories, London, UK

G. Rumsby, G. M. Woodward (eds.), *Disorders of Steroidogenesis*,
https://doi.org/10.1007/978-3-319-96364-8

Androsterone

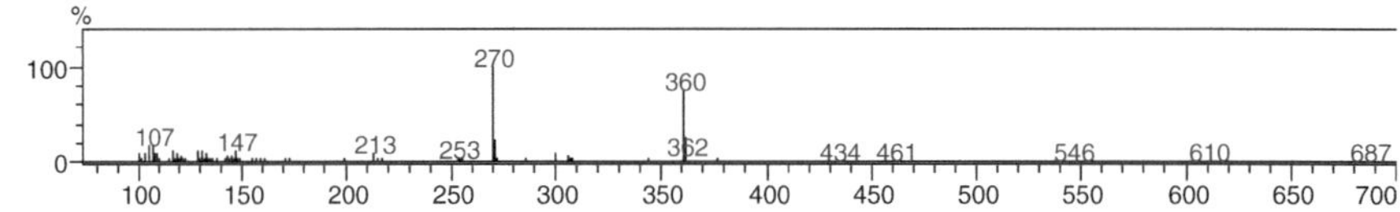

Aetiocholanolone

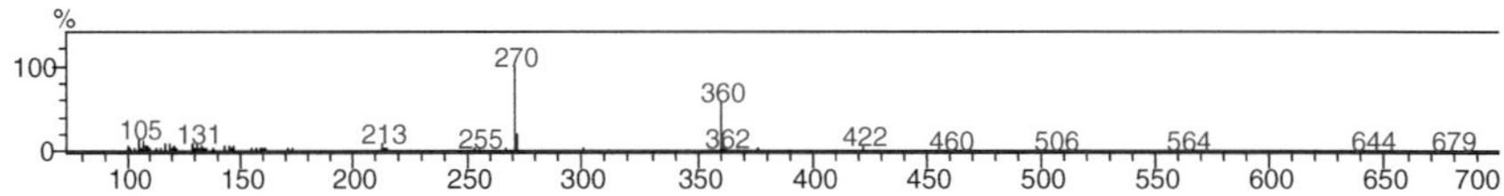

Dehydroepiandrosterone

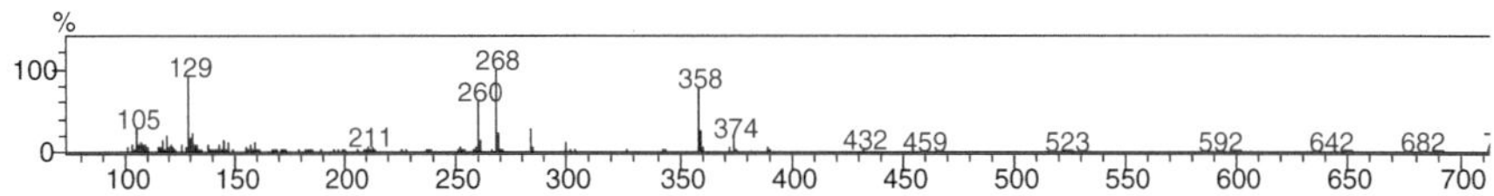

Androstenediol

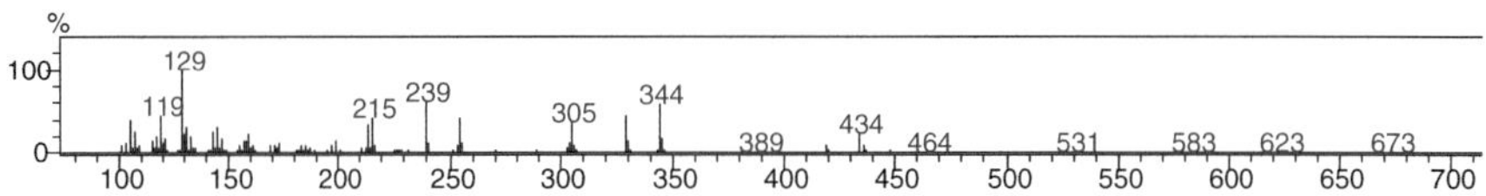

17-Hydroxypregnanolone (peak 1)

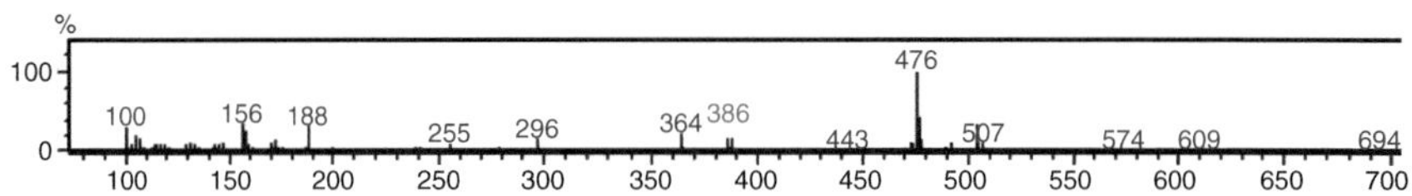

11β-Hydroxyandrosterone

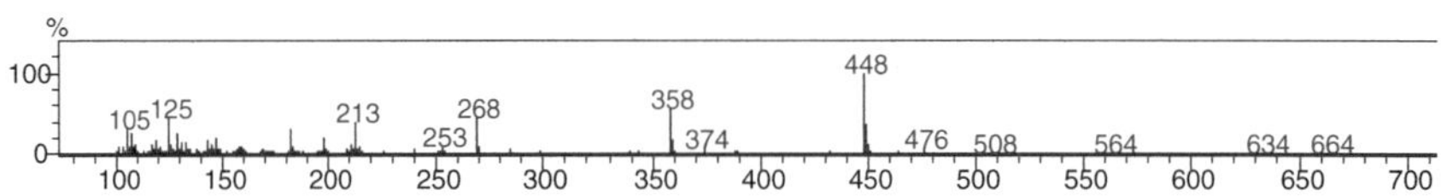

11β-Hydroxyaetiocholanolone

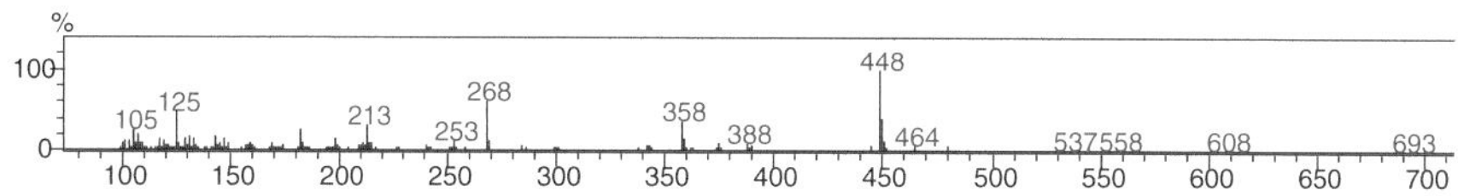

17-Hydroxypregnanolone (peak 2)

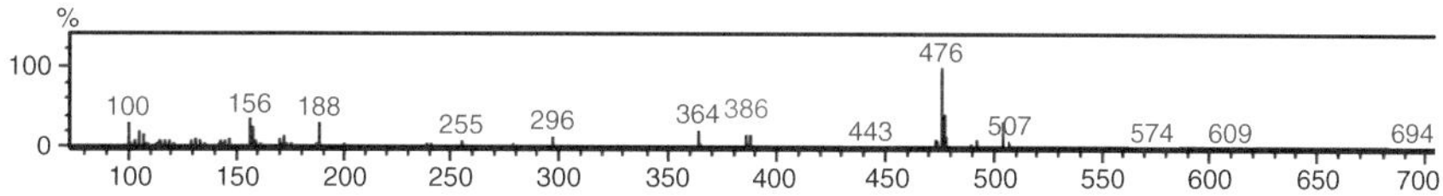

16α-Hydroxydehydroepiandrosterone (two epimers)

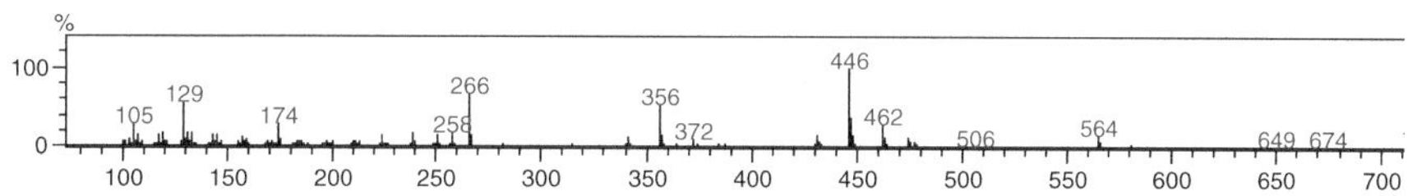

15,17-Dihydroxypregnanolone

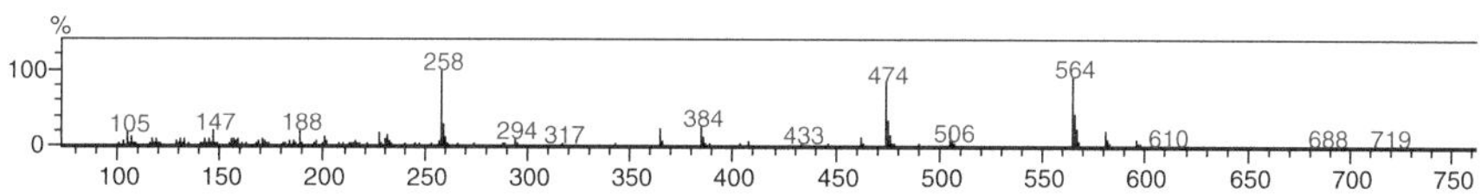

Enterodiol

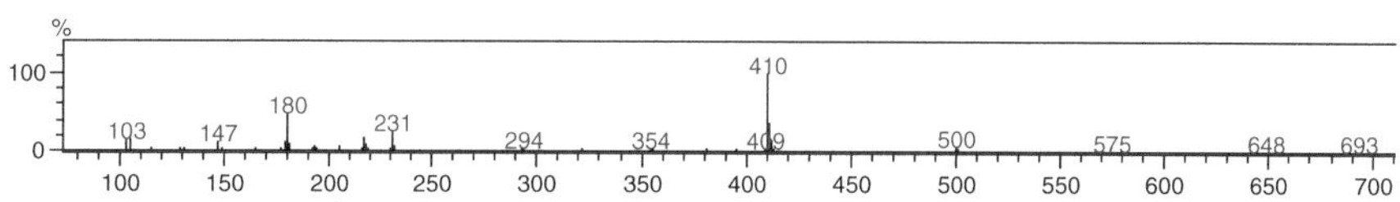

Pregnane-3α,20α-diol

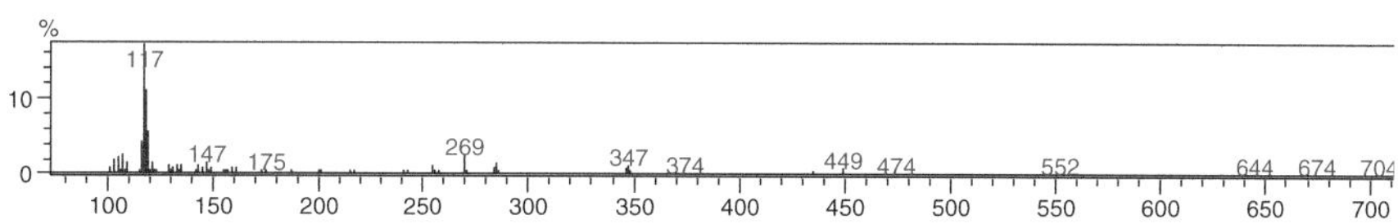

Enterolactone

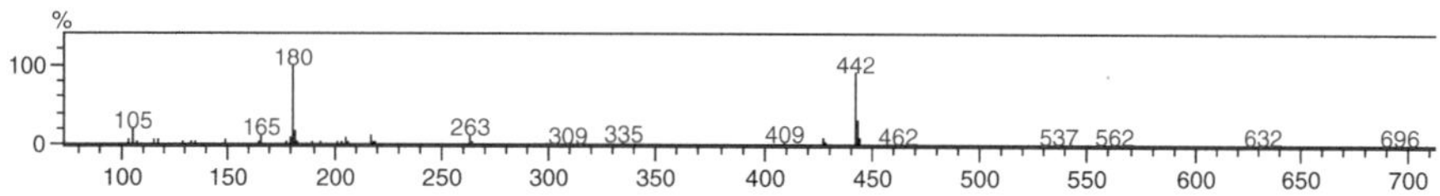

16β-Hydroxydehydroepiandrosterone (two epimers)

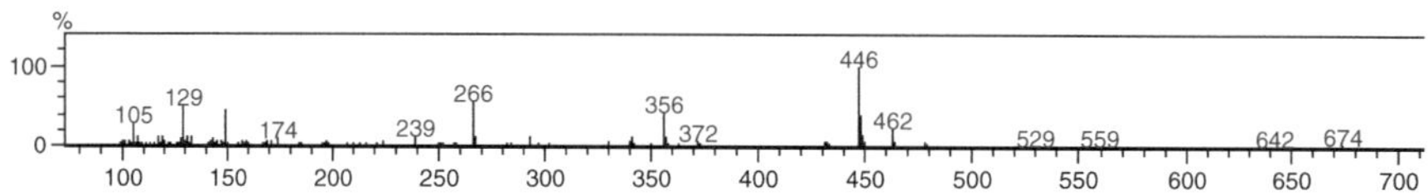

Pregnanetriol

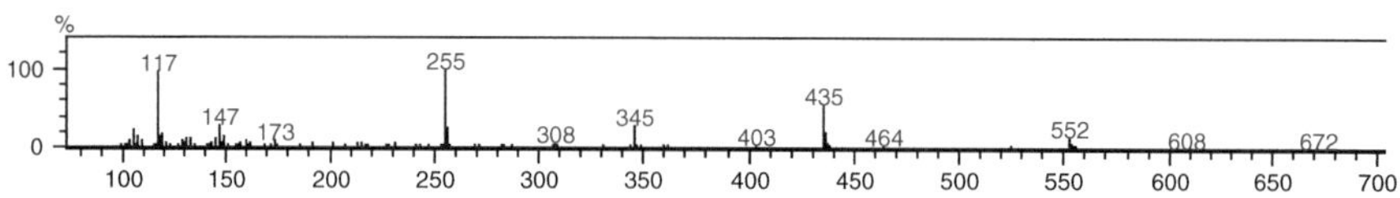

5-Pregnene-3β,20α-diol

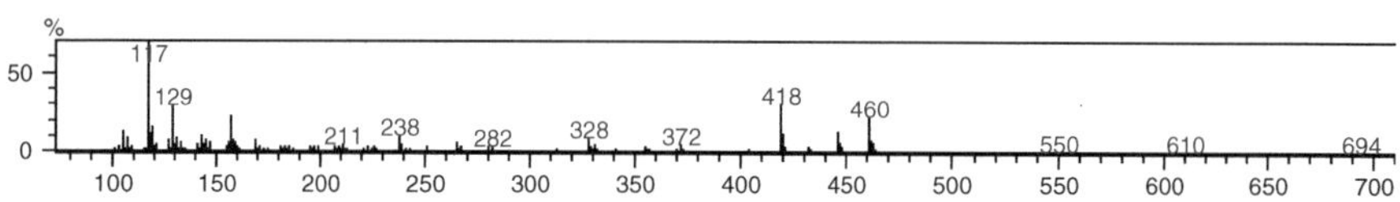

16-Oxoandrostenetriol and 15β,16α-dihydroxydehydroepiandrosterone

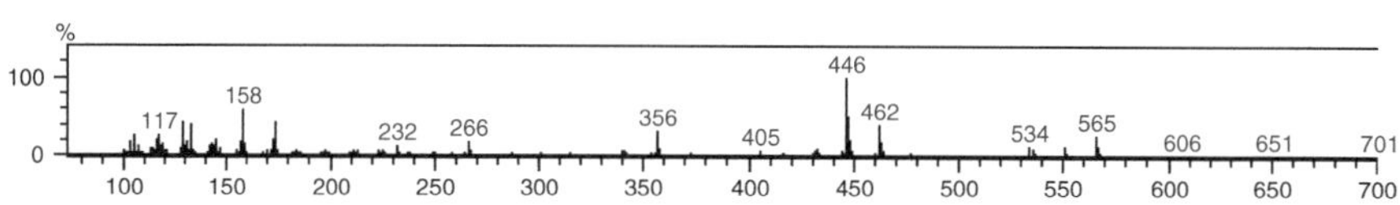

Androstenetriol

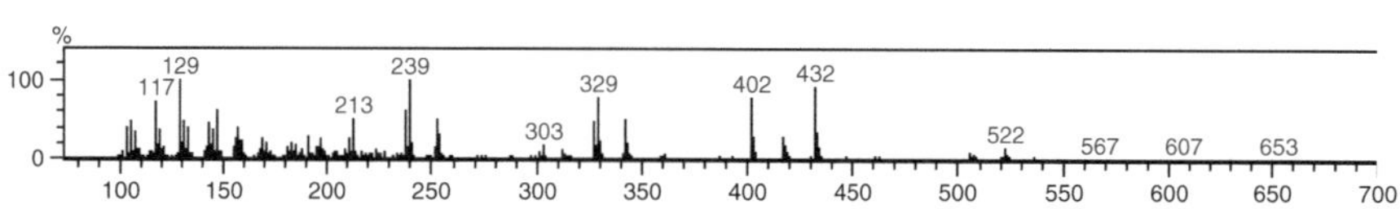

Tetrahydro-11-deoxycortisol

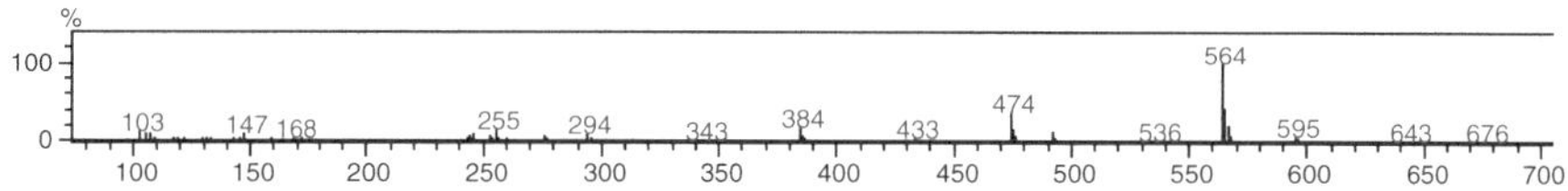

Tetrahydrodeoxycorticosterone (THDOC)

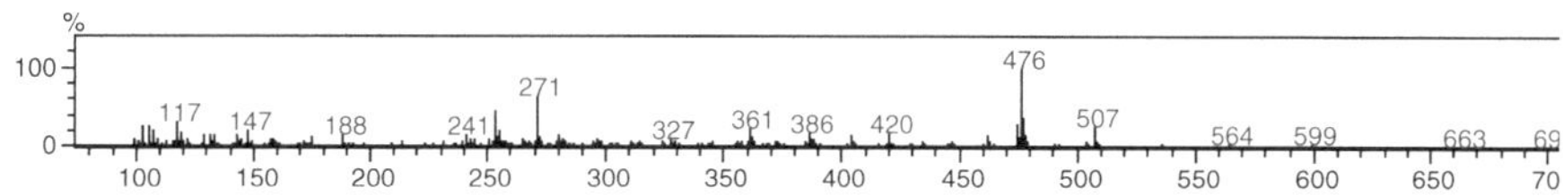

16,18-Dihydroxydehydroepiandrosterone (peak 1)

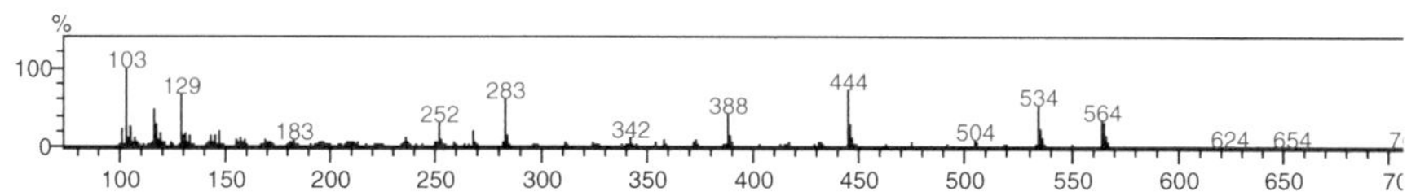

5-Pregnene-3α,16α,20α-triol

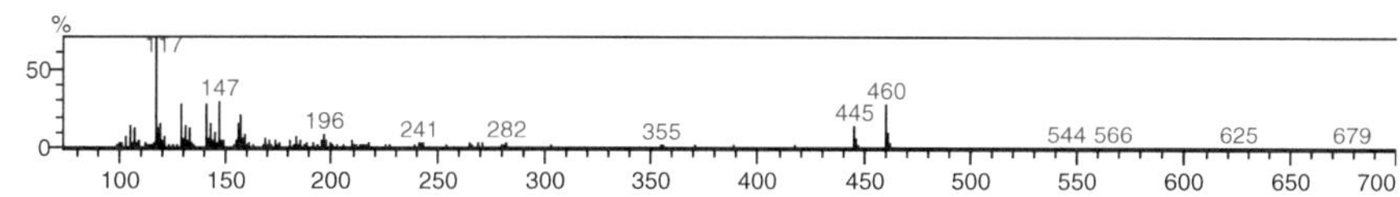

16,18-Dihydroxydehydroepiandrosterone (peak 2)

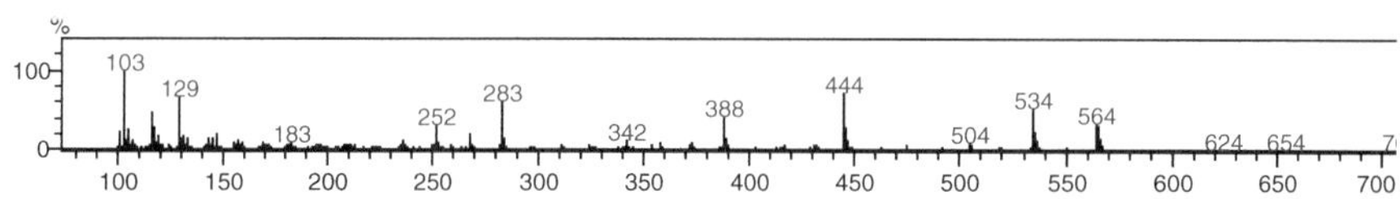

Oestriol

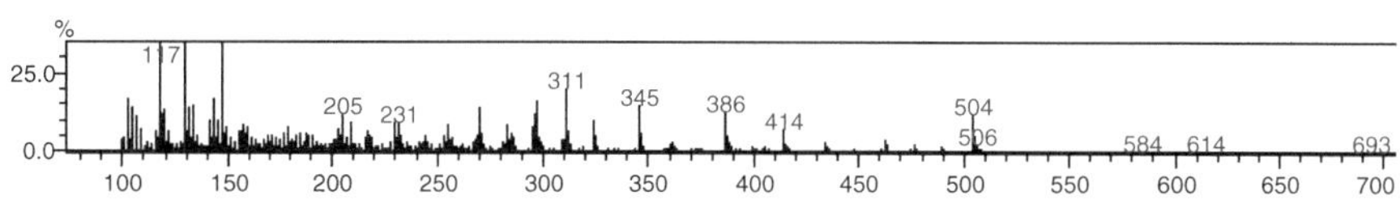

11-Oxopregnanetriol

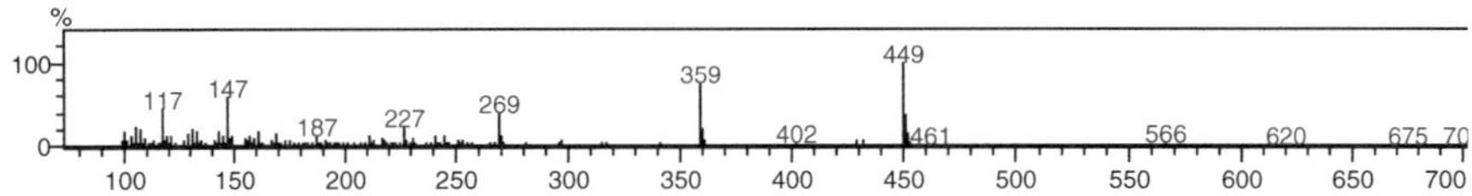

16α-Hydroxypregnenolone

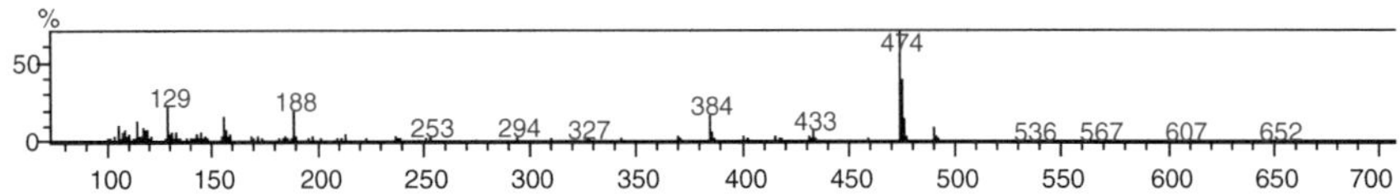

Hexahydro11-deoxycortisol (peak 1)

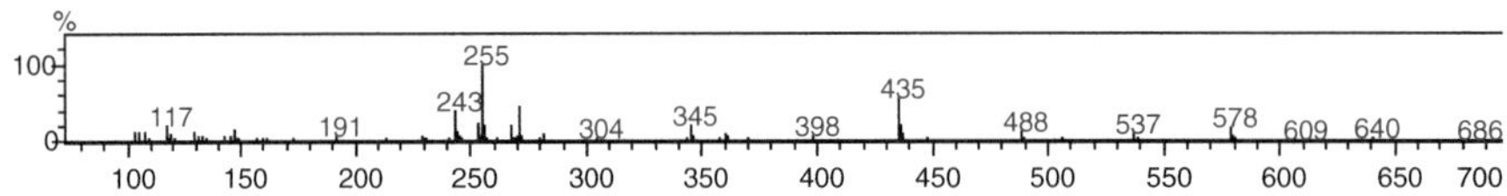

5-Pregnene-3β,17α,20α-triol

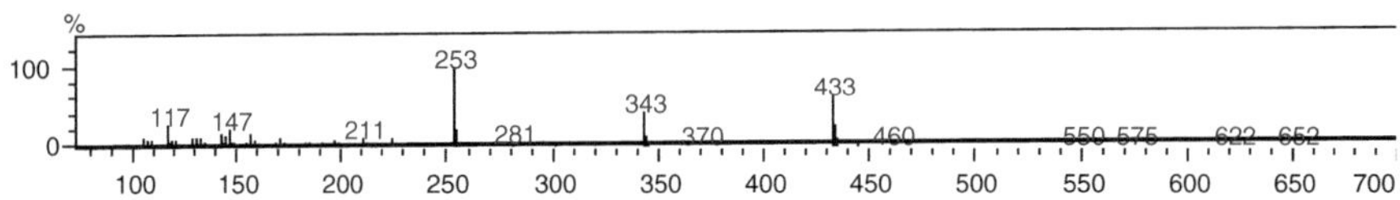

5-Androstene-3β, 15β,16α,17β-tetrol

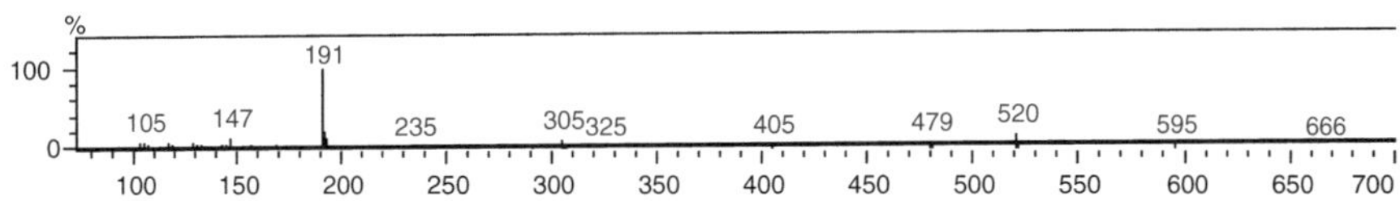

6-Hydroxy-tetrahydro-11-deoxycortisol

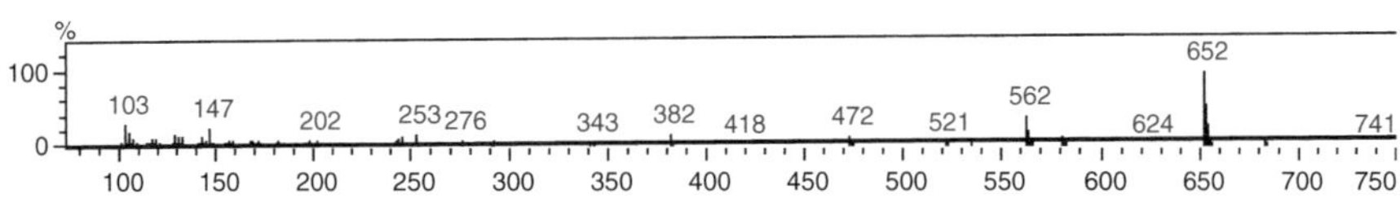

3β,16α-Dihydroxypregnatrien-20-one

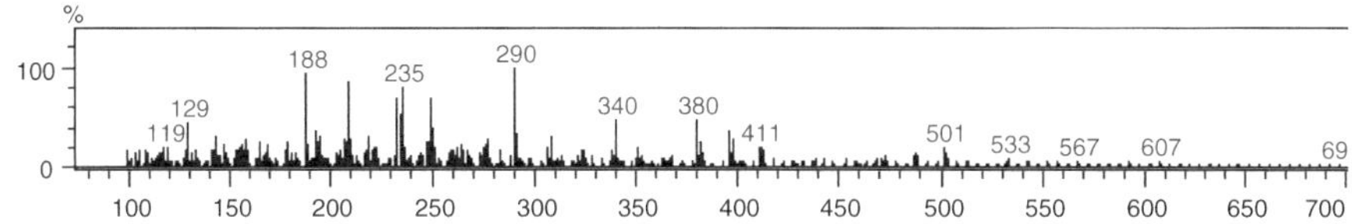

3β,16α-Dihydroxy-5,8(9)-pregnadien-20-one

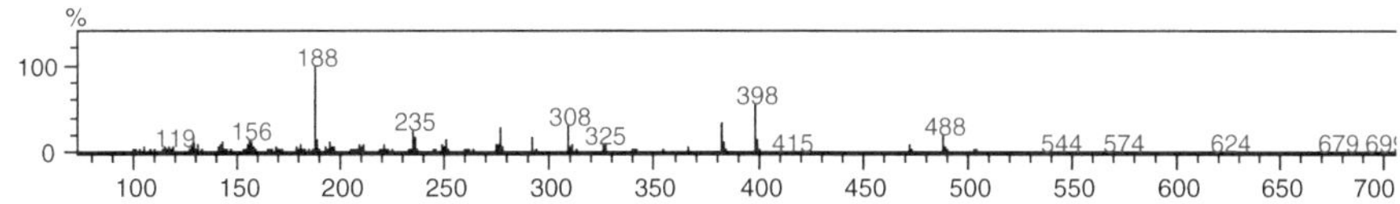

3β,16α-Dihydroxy-5,7-pregnadien-20-one

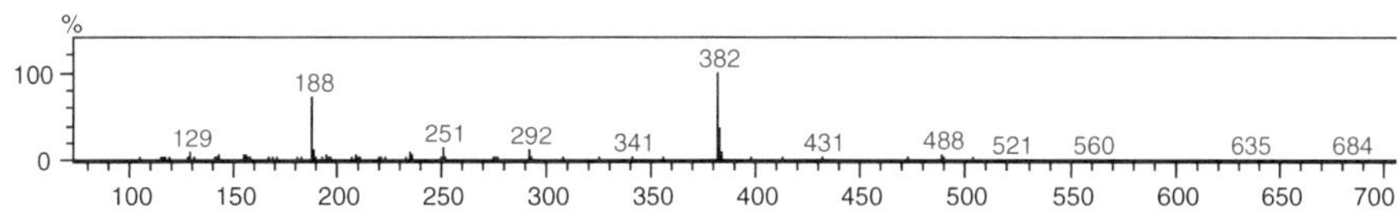

Hexahydro-11-deoxycortisol (peak 1)

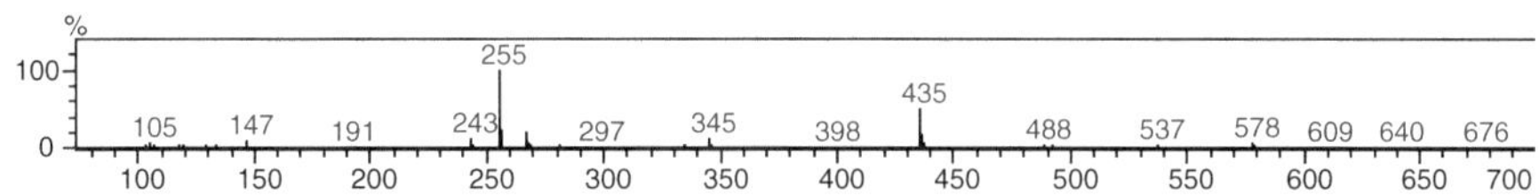

Tetrahydrocortisone (THE)

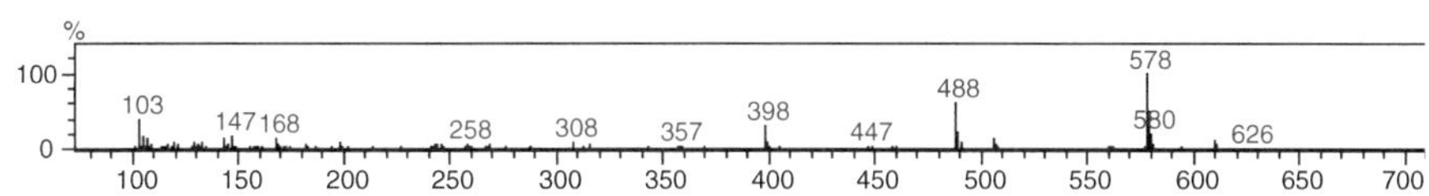

Hexahydro-11-deoxycortisol (peak 2)

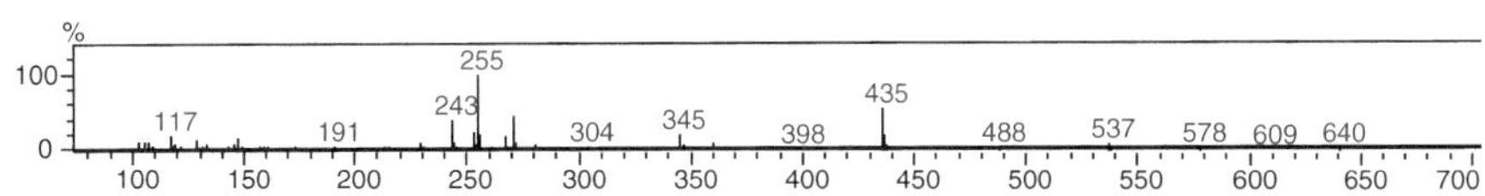

5-Androstene-3β, 15β, 16α,18-tetrol

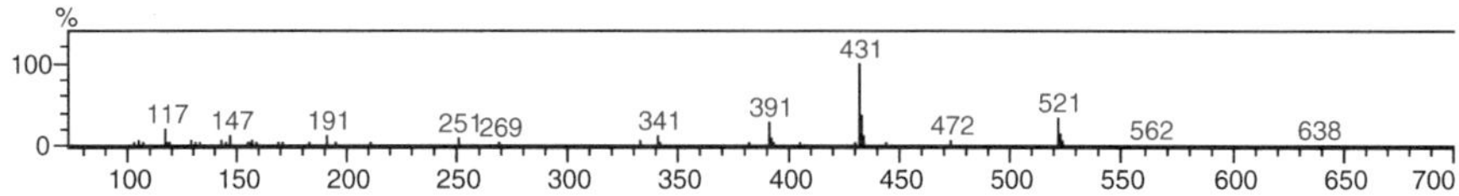

Tetrahydro-11-dehydrocorticosterone (THA)

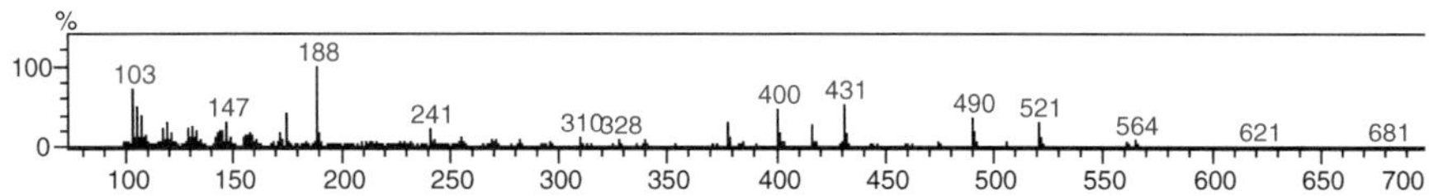

Tetrahydroaldosterone hemiacetal

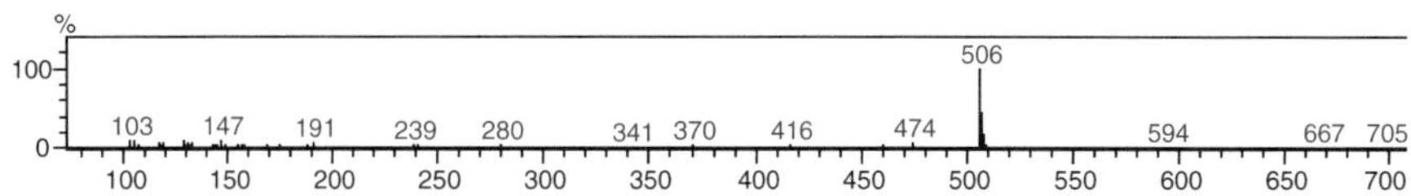

Tetrahydrocorticosterone (THB)

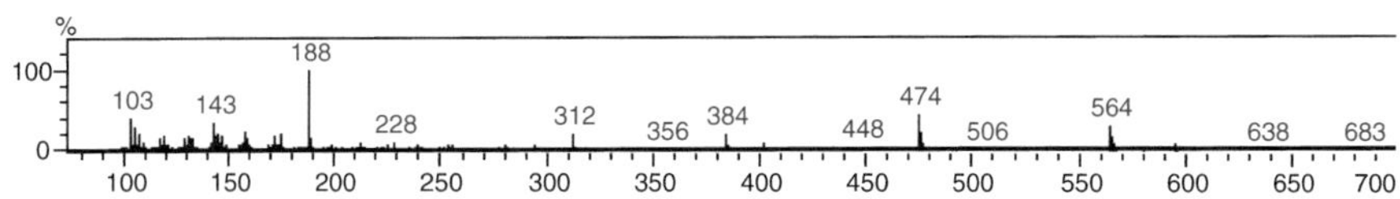

Allo-tetrahydro-11-dehydrocorticosterone (alloTHA)

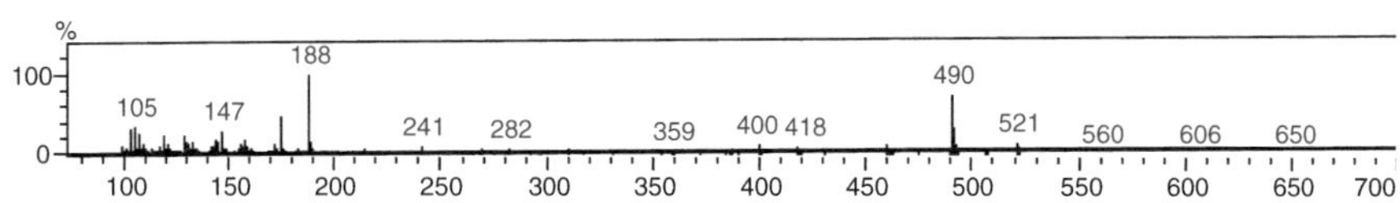

Allo-tetrahydrocorticosterone (alloTHB)

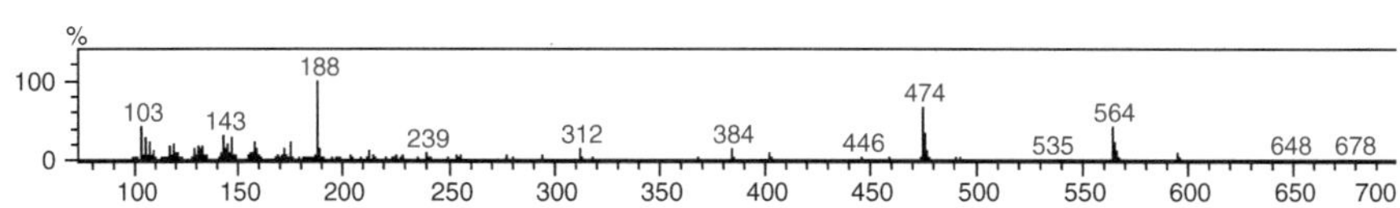

Tetrahydrocortisol (THF)

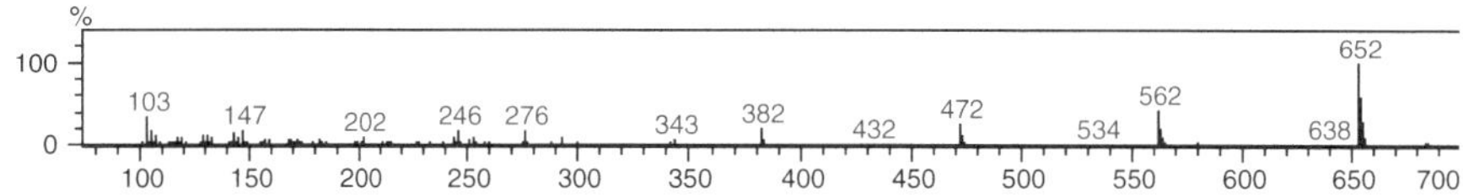

5α-Tetrahydrocortisol (5α-THF)

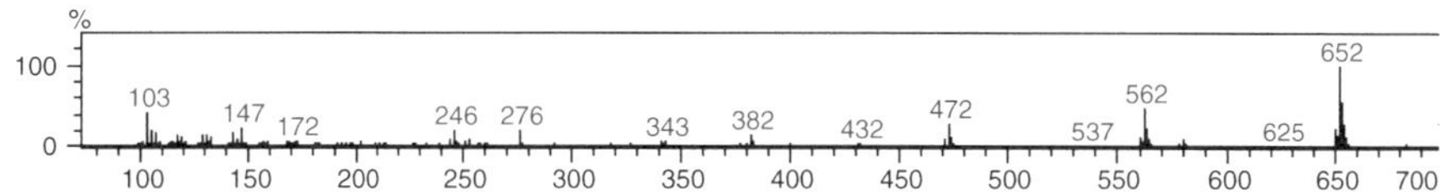

α-Cortolone

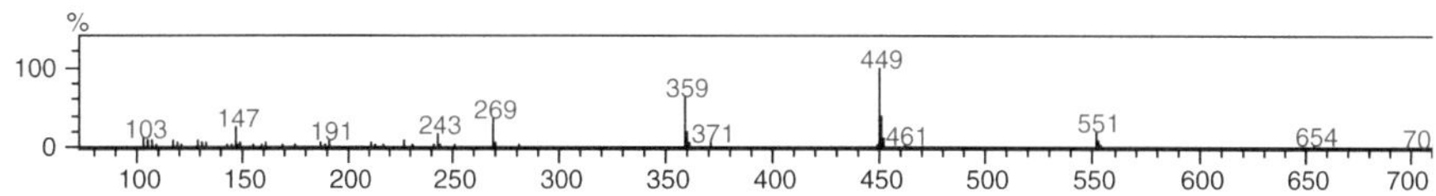

18-Hydroxy-11-dehydrocorticosterone (18OH THA)

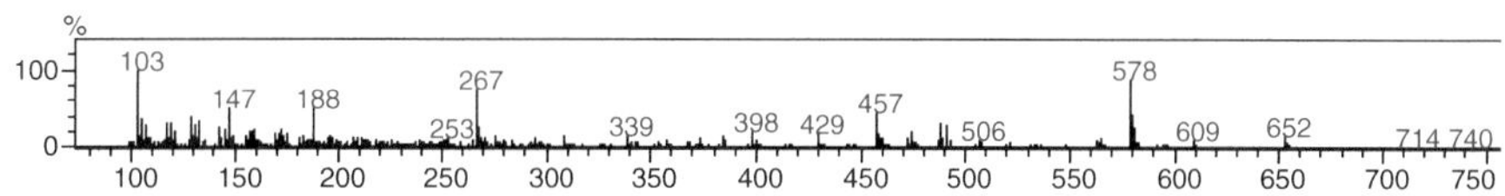

β-Cortolone, β-cortol

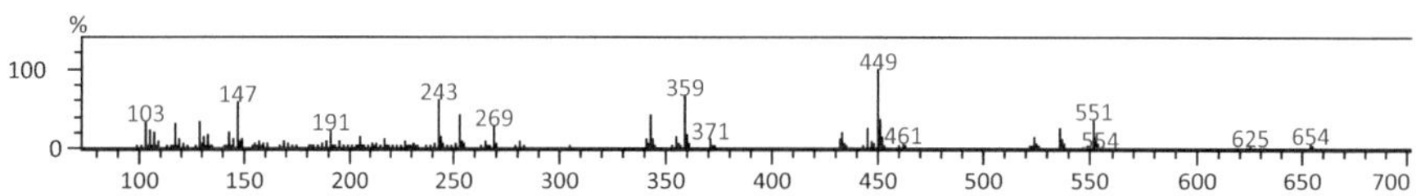

Hexahydro-11-dehydrocorticosterone (HHA 20α)

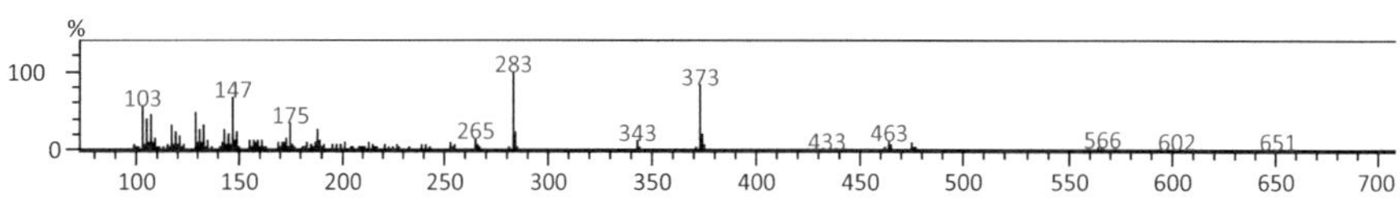

Hexahydro-11-hydroxycorticosterone (HHB)

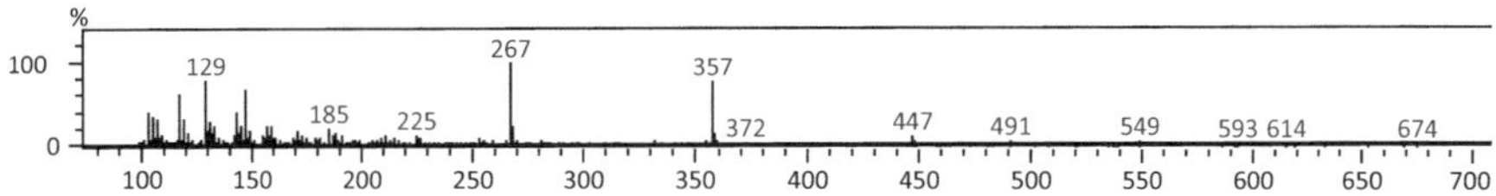

6α-Hydroxy THE

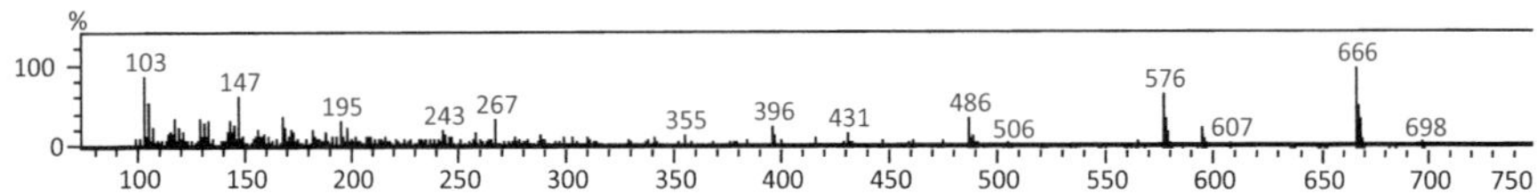

6α-Hydroxytetrahydro-11-dehydrocorticosterone (6αOH THA)

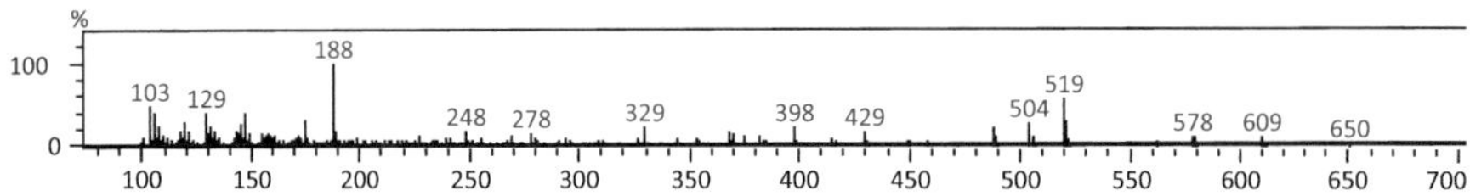

18-Hydroxy tetrahydrocorticosterone (18OH THB)

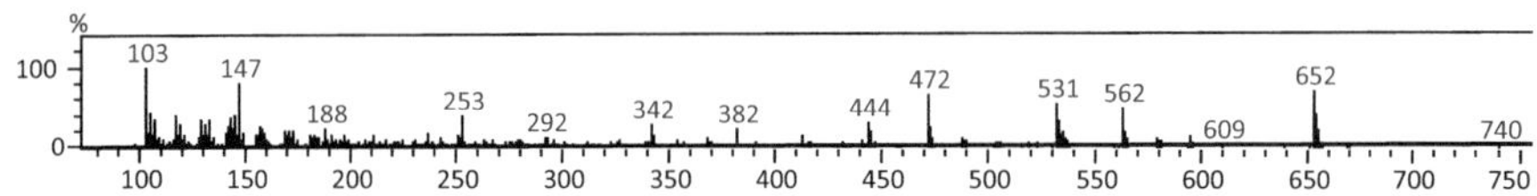

Cholesterol

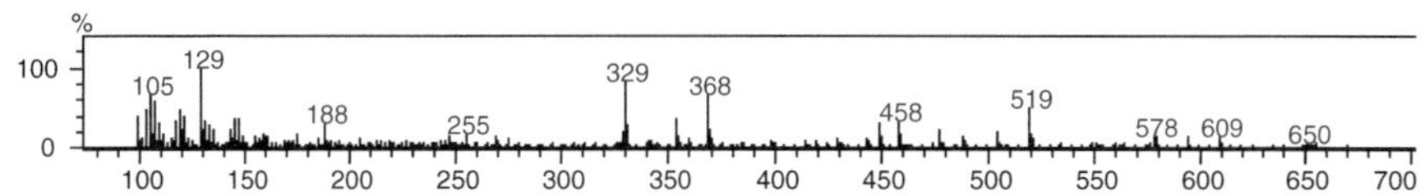

Tetrahydroaldosterone

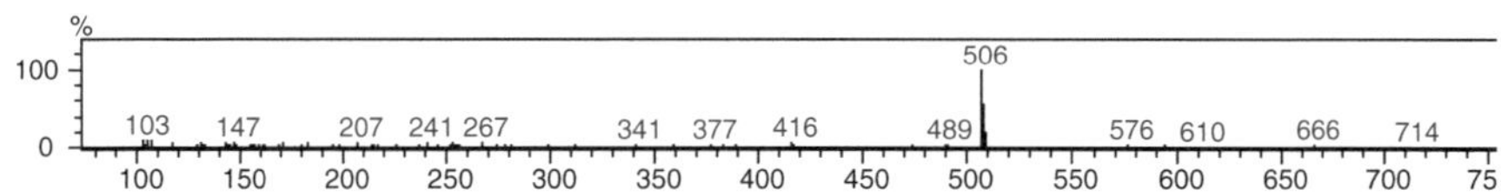

Hexahydro-tetrahydrocorticosterone (HHB)

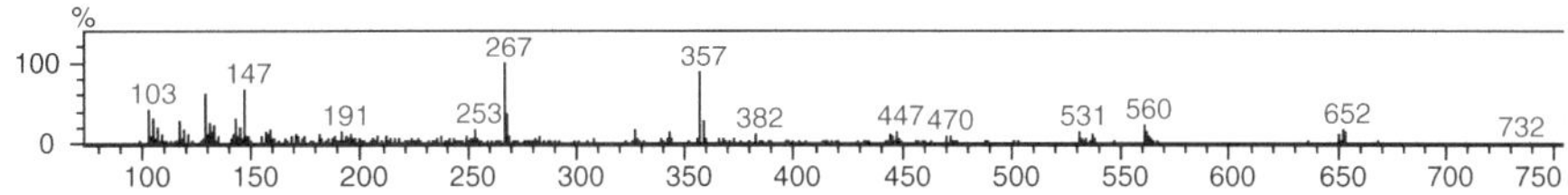

α-Cortol

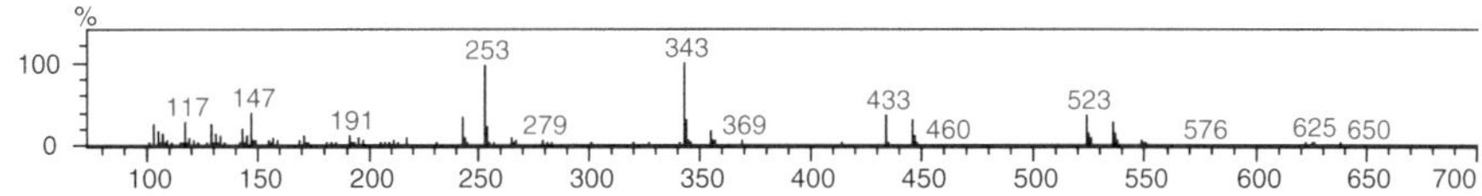

6α-Hydroxy-20α-cortolone

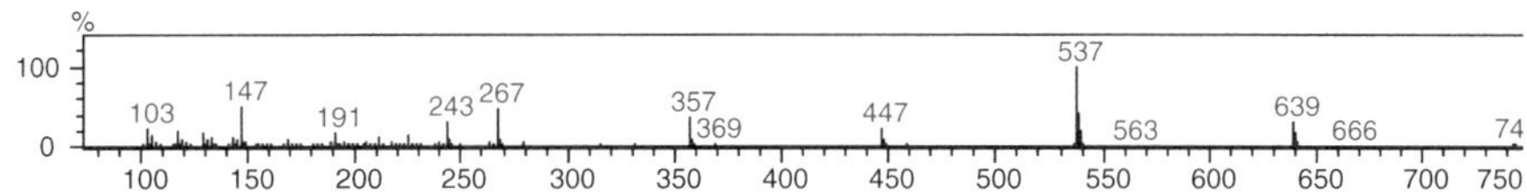

6α-Hydroxy-20β-cortolone

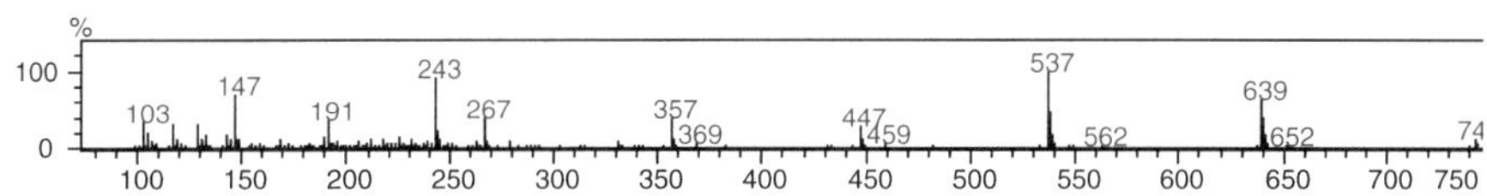

1β-Hydroxy-20β-cortolone

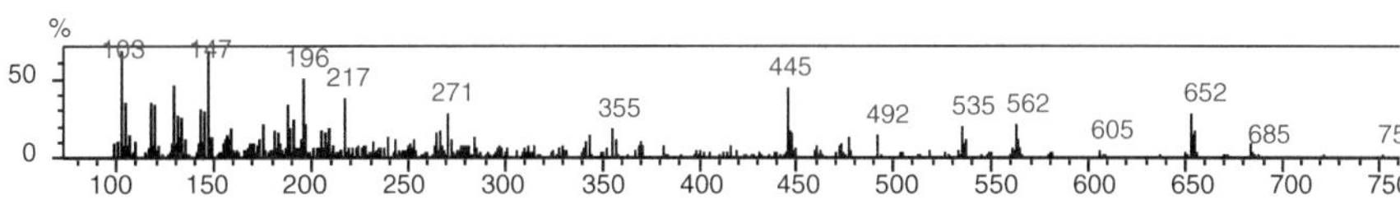

Stigmasterol

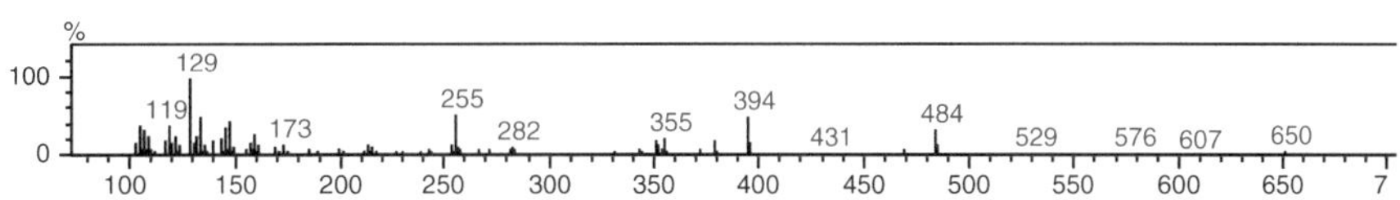

3β,16α,17α-Trihydroxy-5α pregnane-7,20-dione ('607')

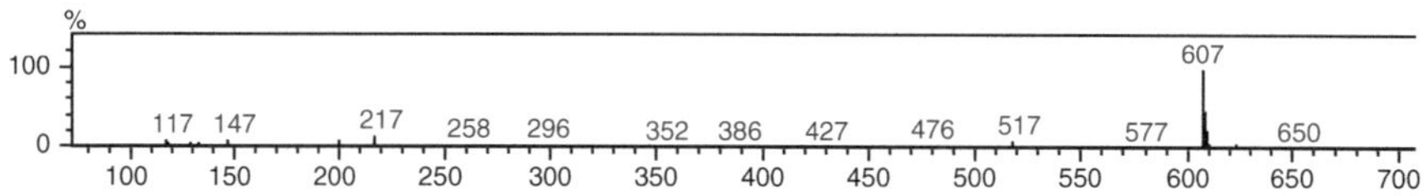

Prednisolone

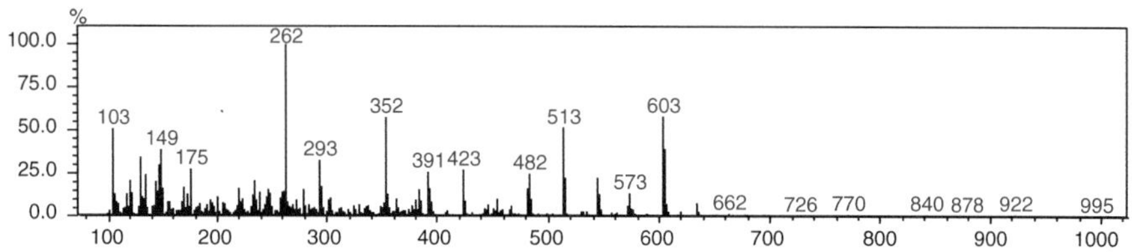

6-Hydroxyprednisolone

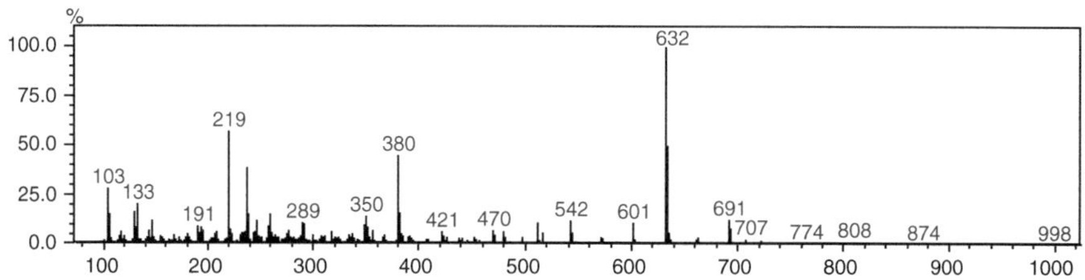

Cortisol (two peaks)

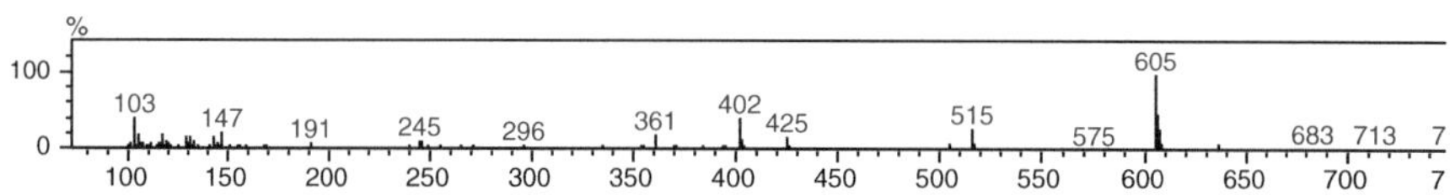

18-Hydroxycortisol

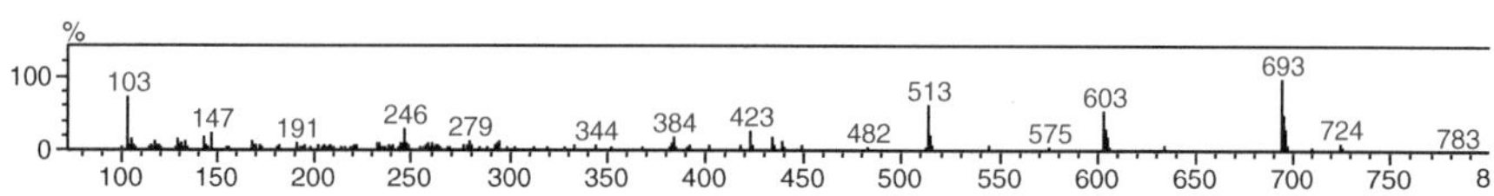

6β-Hydroxycortisol

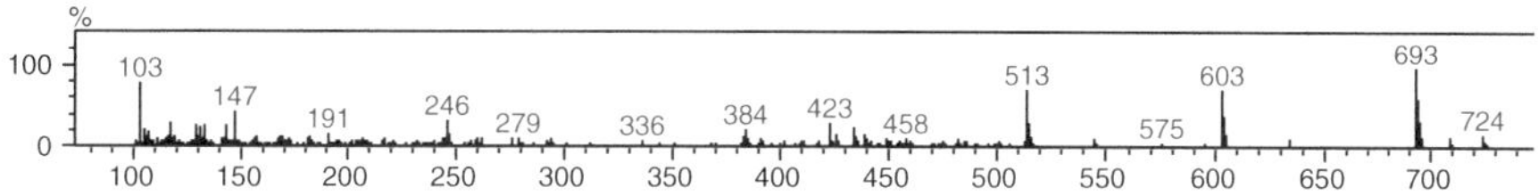

Cholesteryl butyrate (internal standard)

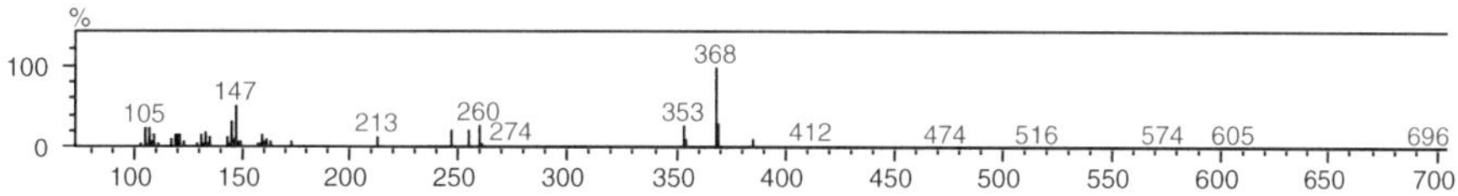

Index

G. Rumsby, G. M. Woodward (eds.), *Disorders of Steroidogenesis*,
https://doi.org/10.1007/978-3-319-96364-8

I

T

U

V

W

MIX
Papier aus verantwortungsvollen Quellen
Paper from responsible sources
FSC® C105338

If you have any concerns about our products,
you can contact us on
ProductSafety@springernature.com

In case Publisher is established outside the EU,
the EU authorized representative is:
Springer Nature Customer Service Center GmbH
Europaplatz 3, 69115 Heidelberg, Germany

Printed by Libri Plureos GmbH
in Hamburg, Germany